TABLE OF C

GENERAL SURGERY	2
OTHOPEDIC SURGERY	42
VASCULAR SURGERY	64
NEURO-SPINE SURGERY	97
GYN SURGERY	115
PLASTIC AND COSMETIC SURGERY	130
ENT SURGERY	154
INDEX	182

THANK YOU FOR PURCHASING LEARNING SURGICAL INSTRUMENTS. WITHIN THESE PAGES YOU WILL FIND THE INSTRUMENTS YOU NEED TO KNOW TO GET OFF ON THE RIGHT FOOT IN THE OPERATING ROOM FROM DAY ONE. YOU WILL FIND THERE IS A LIFE TIME OF LEARNING TO BE HAD IN THE OPERATING ROOM. IT HAS BEEN OUR GOAL TO HELP INDIVIDUALS LEARN THE BASICS WITHOUT AN OVERWHELMING AMOUNT OF DETAIL.

JAMES NIDEFFER RN, BSN
ELIZABETH NIDEFFER RN, MSN

GENERAL SURGERY

10 Blade

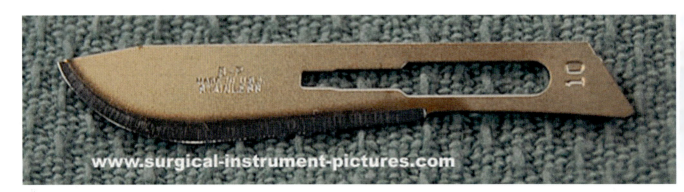

Surgical Instrument: 10 Blade
Alias: Skin Blade
Use: For making the skin incision
Additional Info: Attaches to a #3 Handle

15 Blade

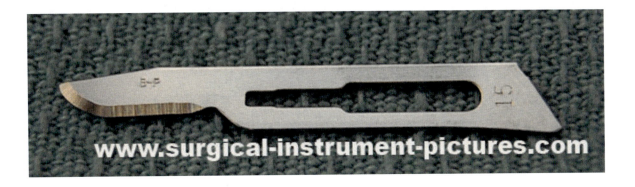

Surgical Instrument: 15 Blade
Alias: None
Use: Multi-purpose blade
Additional Info: Used on the #3 or #7 Handle

11 Blade

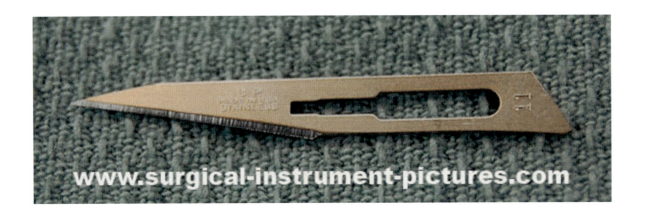

Surgical Instrument: 11 Blade
Alias: None
Use: Cutting
Additional Info: Used for making incisions for laparoscopic trocars

#3 Knife Handle ~~*~~ old

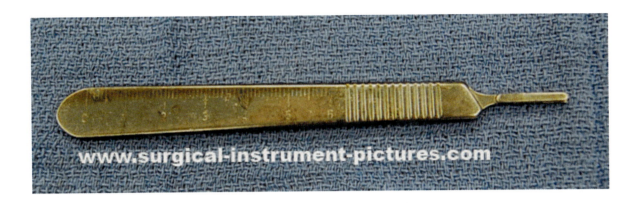

Surgical Instrument: #3 Knife Handle
Alias: Scalpel
Use: Holds a knife blade
Additional Info: Used with the 10, 11, and 15 Blades

#7 Knife Handle & ENT

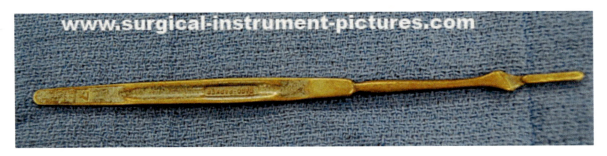

Surgical Instrument: #7 Knife Handle
Alias: None
Use: For attaching a knife blade
Additional Info: Use with a 15 Blade

Adson Forceps

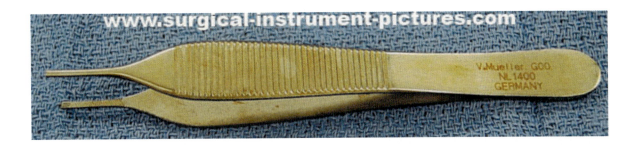

Surgical Instrument: Adson Forceps
Alias: Skin Forceps
Use: Grasping
Additional Info: Common forcep for use in skin suturing

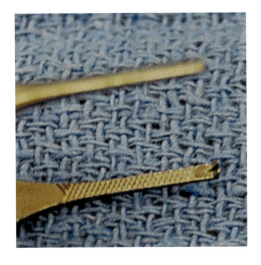

Adson Brown Forceps

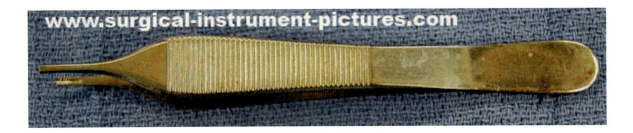

Surgical Instrument: Adson Brown Forceps
Alias: None
Use: Grasping
Additional Info: Differentiated from regular Adsons by the teeth. Commonly used in cosmetic and ENT surgery

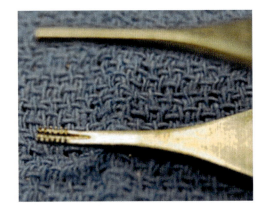

Bonney Forceps

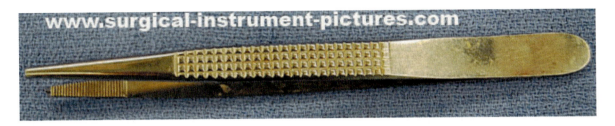

Surgical Instrument: Bonney Forceps
Alias: Bonneys
Use: Grasping
Additional Info: Heavy pickup used for grasping the fascia to close the peritoneum

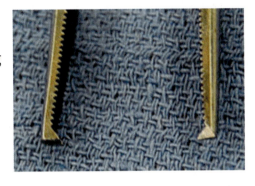

Debakey Forceps

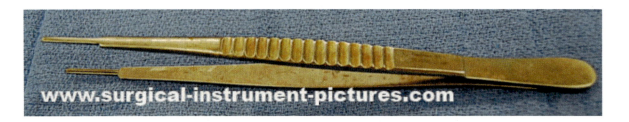

Surgical Instrument: Debakey Forceps
Alias: None
Use: Grasping
Additional Info: Used to grasp more delicate structures such as vessels, bowel and soft tissue

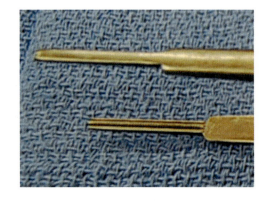

Pick up w/ teeth
Rat Tooth Forceps

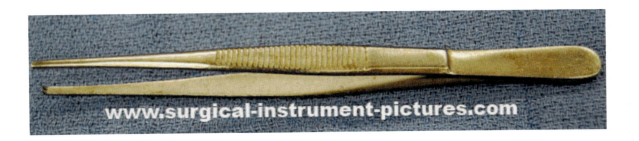

Surgical Instrument: Rat Tooth Forceps
Alias: Toothed Pick Ups
Use: Grasping
Additional Info: Commonly used to grasp bone or when closing the belly button site for laparoscopic surgery

Russian Forceps

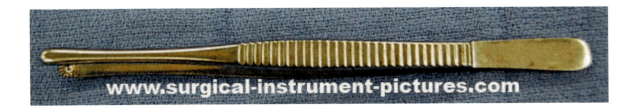

Surgical Instrument: Russian Forceps
Alias: None
Use: Grasping
Additional Info: Non-traumatic multi-purpose grasper

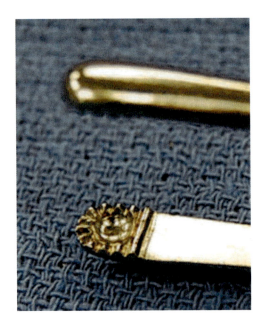

Allis Clamp

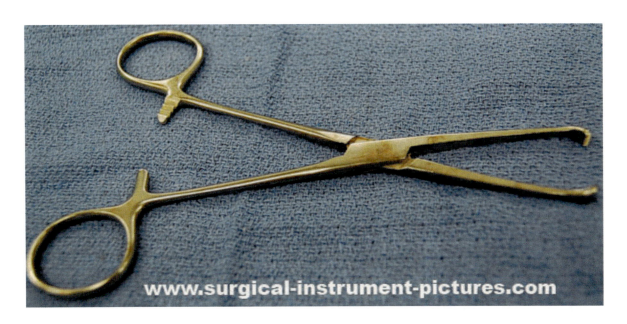

Surgical Instrument: Allis
Alias: None
Use: Grasping
Additional Info: For grasping soft tissue

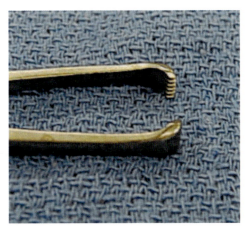

Babcock Clamp

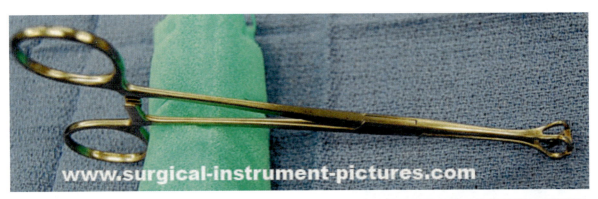

Surgical Instrument: Babcock
Alias: None
Use: Grasping
Additional Info: For grasping soft tissue, lymph nodes and bowel tissue

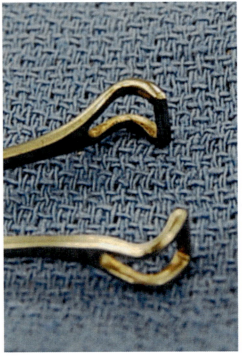

Carmault Clamp / Mayo

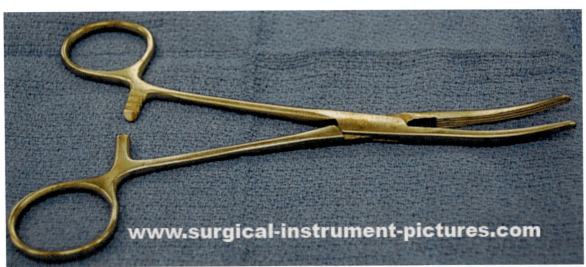

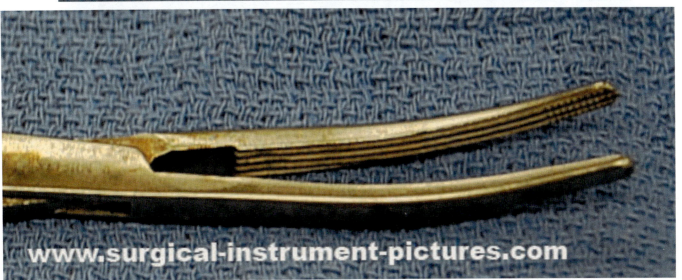

Surgical Instrument: Carmault
Alias: None
Use: Clamp
Additional Info: Larger than a kelly and the same size as a peon, the Carmault with its characteristic jaws are used to clamp bowel.

Kelly Clamp

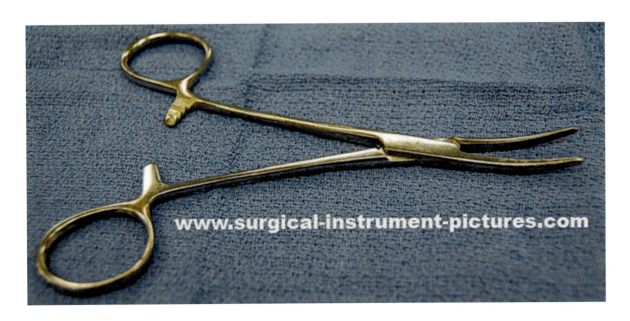

Surgical Instrument: Kelly
Alias: Snap
Use: Clamping
Additional Info: The most basic of the clamps, multi-purpose

Mosquito Clamp

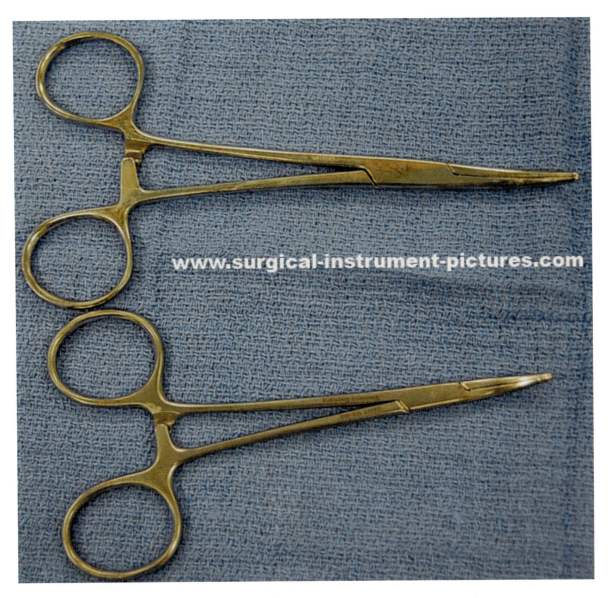

Surgical Instrument: Mosquito Clamp
Alias: None
Use: Clamping, dissection
Additional Info: Smaller than the kelly pictured above, the mosquito has a similar jaw.

Right Angle Clamp

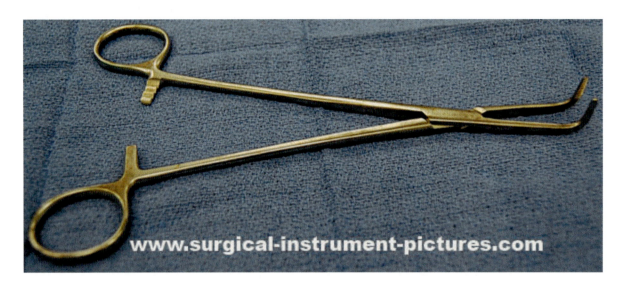

Surgical Instrument: Right Angle
Alias: None
Use: Clamping
Additional Info: Often used to pass things under structures or separate and dissect soft tissue structures

Ring Sponge Forceps

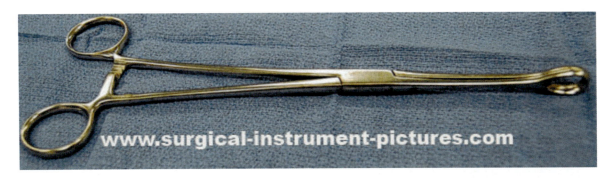

Surgical Instrument: Sponge Forceps
Alias: Sponge stick
Use: Grasping
Additional Info: Often has a ratex folded in the jaw for blunt dissection and dabbing in open abdominal surgeries

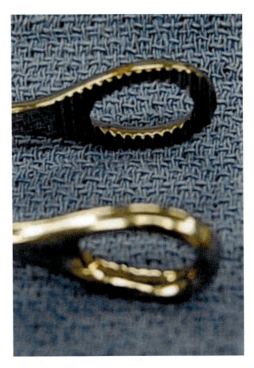

Burlisher
Schnit

Tonsil Clamp

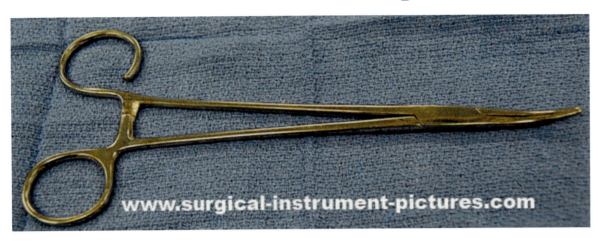

Surgical Instrument: Tonsil
Alias: Schnitt
Use: Clamping
Additional Info: Often used with silk or vicryl ties off the end for ligating structures

Towel Clamp

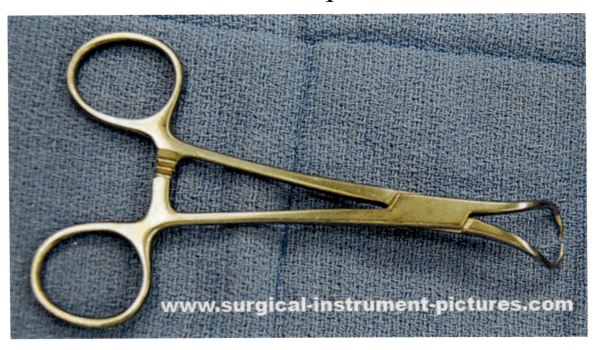

Surgical Instrument: Towel Clamp
Alias: None
Use: Grasping and approximating
Additional Info: None

Non Perforating Towel Clamp

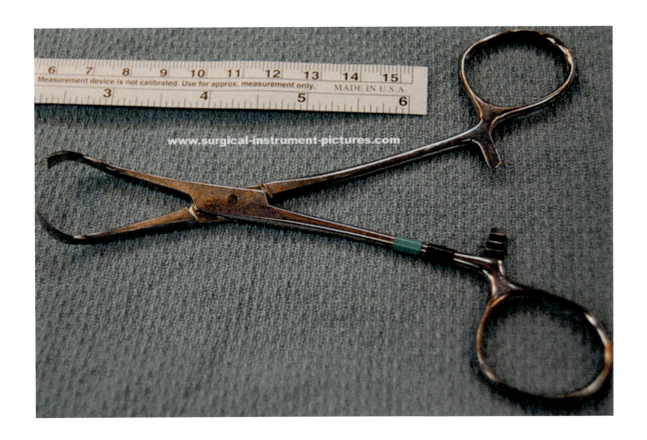

Surgical Instrument: Non-perforating towel clamp
Alias: Non-penetrating towel clamp
Use: Grasping
Additional Info: Often used to clamp surgical drapes

Army-Navy Retractors

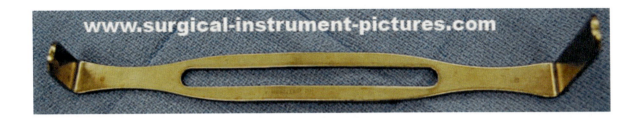

Surgical Instrument: Army-Navy
Alias: US Retractor
Use: Retraction
Additional Info: None

Deaver Retractor

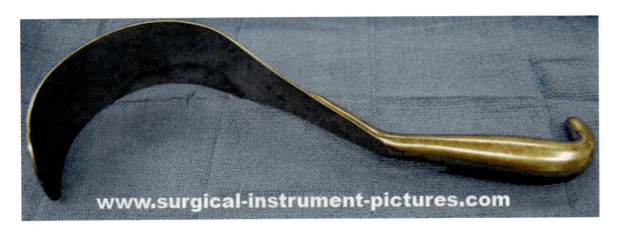

Surgical Instrument: Deaver
Alias: None
Use: Retraction
Additional Info: Available in a variety of widths

Senn Retractor

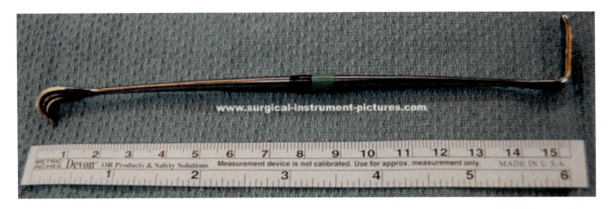

Surgical Instrument: Senn Retractor
Alias: Senn Rake
Use: Retraction
Additional Info: Available and pictured with both sharp and dull teeth

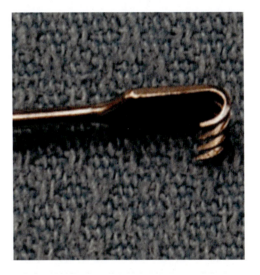

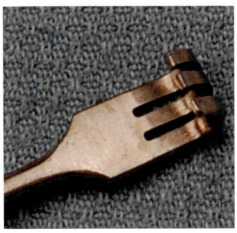

Goelet Retractor

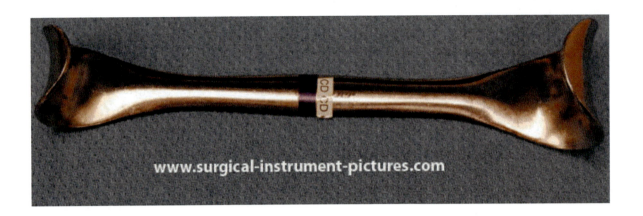

Surgical Instrument: Goelet
Alias: None
Use: Retraction
Additional Info: None

Isreal Retractor

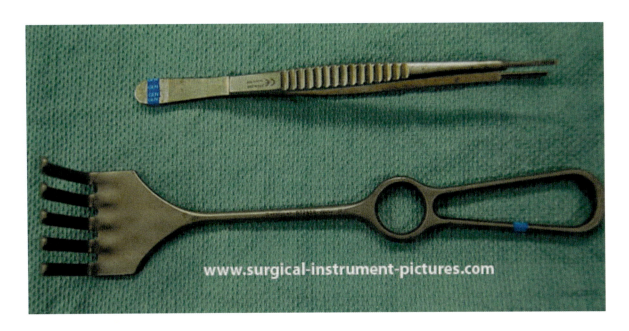

Surgical Instrument: Isreal
Alias: None
Use: Retraction
Additional Info: Pictured below a debakey

Bodywall Retractor

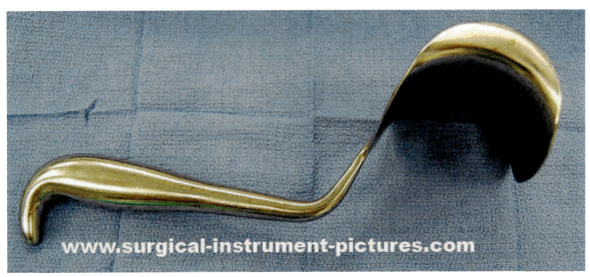

Surgical Instrument: Mayo Bodywall Retractor
Alias: None
Use: Retraction
Additional Info: Used for large open abdominal surgeries

Richardson Retractor

Finger Rich /A&P

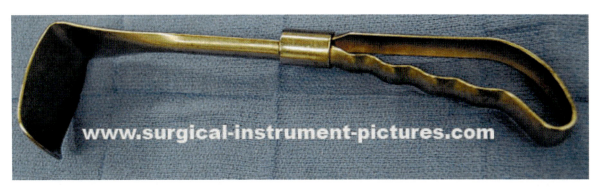

Surgical Instrument: Richardson
Alias: Rich
Use: Retraction
Additional Info: Common retractor available both double and single ended as well as in a variety of sizes

Weitlaner Retractor

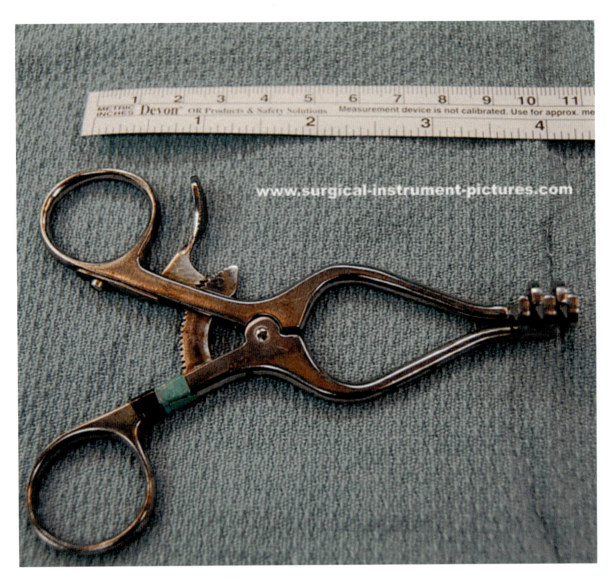

Surgical Instrument: Weitlaner
Alias: Self Retainer
Use: Retraction
Additional Info: This self-retaining retractor is available in a variety of sizes and with sharp or dull teeth

Sharp Weitlaner Retractor

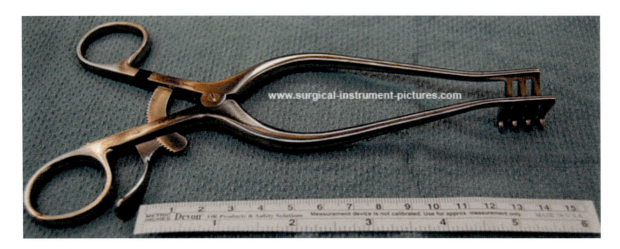

Surgical Instrument: Sharp Weitlaner
Alias: Weety
Use: Retraction
Additional Info: Often miss-pronounced "wheatlander"

Curved Mayo Scissors

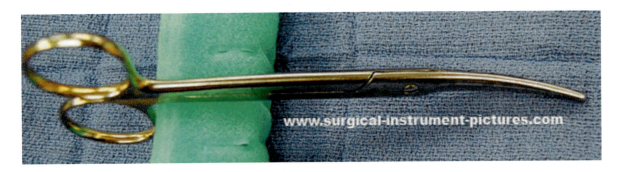

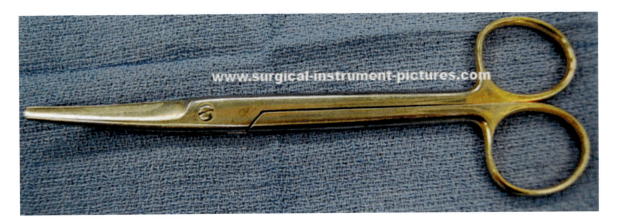

Surgical Instrument: Curved Mayo Scissors
Alias: Curved Mayos
Use: Cutting
Additional Info: Larger then Metz often used for cutting tough tissue

Mayo Scissors

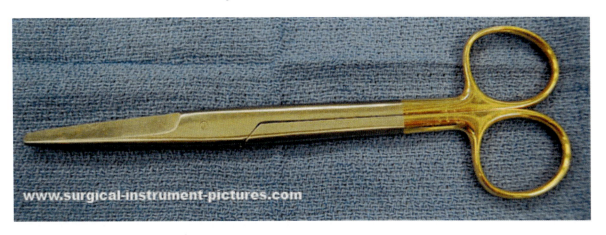

Surgical Instrument: Mayo Scissors
Alias: Suture Scissors
Use: Cutting
Additional Info: Multi-purpose scissor, most often used for cutting suture

Metzenbaum Scissors

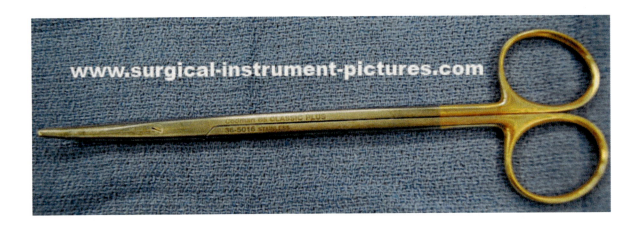

Surgical Instrument: Metzenbaum
Alias: Metz
Use: Cutting
Additional Info: For cutting tissue

Electrocautery Pencil

Green & white

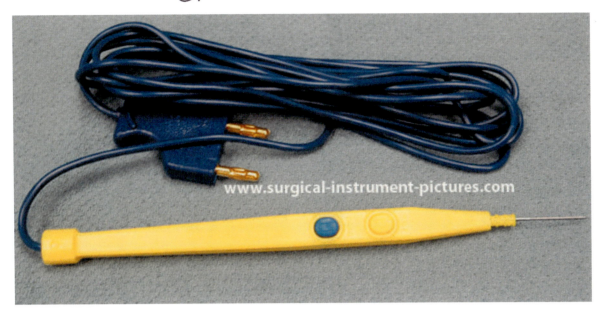

Surgical Instrument: Electrocautery Pencil
Alias: Bovie
Use: Cutting and coagulation
Additional Info: Plugs into an electro surgical unit (ESU) for cutting and coagulation of tissue. Requires a grounding pad for the patient

Poole Suction

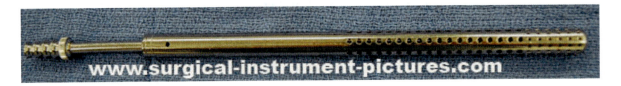

Surgical Instrument: Poole Suction
Alias: None
Use: Suction
Additional Info: Used for suction of large volumes of irrigation fluid out of the abdominal cavity

Yankauer Suction Tip

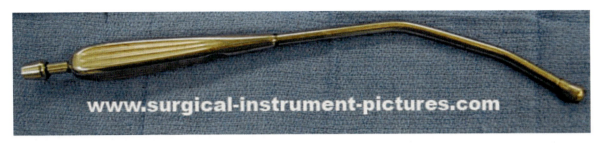

Surgical Instrument: Yankauer Suction
Alias: None
Use: Suction
Additional Info: Common general surgical suction tip for suctioning of blood and fluid during surgery

Mayo-Hegar Needle Holder

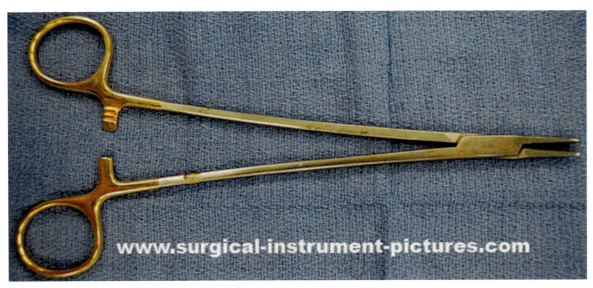

Surgical Instrument: Mayo-Hegar Needle Holder
Alias: Needle Driver
Use: Suturing
Additional Info: Available in a variety of sizes depending on the size of the needle to be used

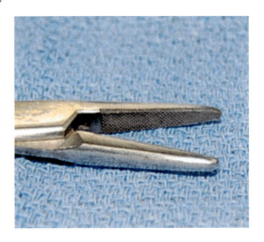

Laparoscopic Trocar and Port

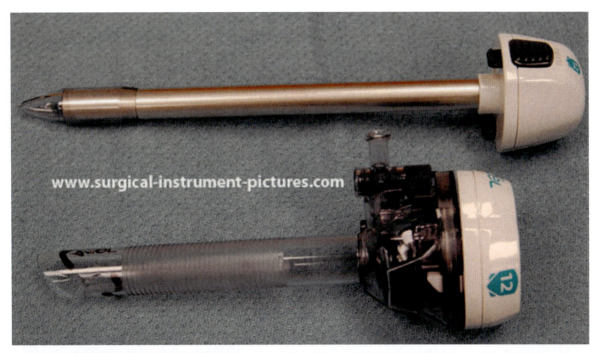

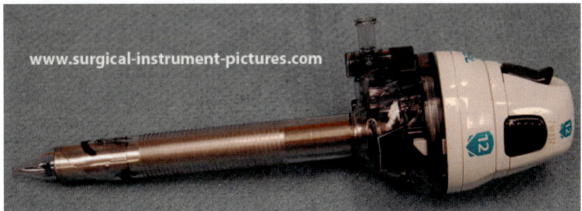

Surgical Instrument: Laparoscopic Trocar
Alias: None
Use: Access for laparoscopic surgery
Additional Info: The trocar is used for introduction of the port to the abdomen but then removed to allow instruments to be passed though

Laparoscopic Grasper

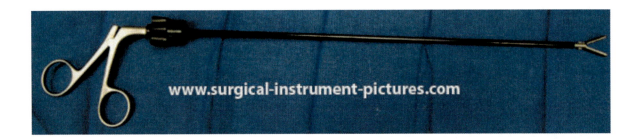

Surgical Instrument: Grasper
Alias: Debakey Grasped
Use: Grasping
Additional Info: For grasping bowel in laparoscopic surgery

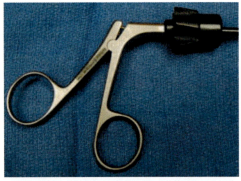

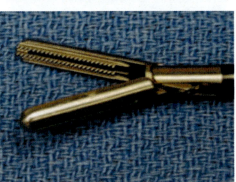

hunters / Debakees

Curved Dissector Maryland

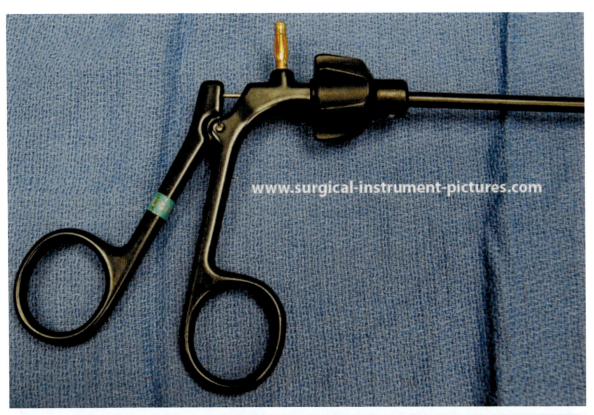

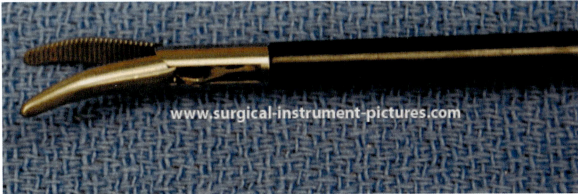

Surgical Instrument: Curved Dissector
Alias: Maryland Grasper, dolphin nose
Use: Dissection
Additional Info: Can be attached to a cautery cord and often is used to ligate vessels and dissect during cholecystectomy surgery

ORTHOPEDIC SURGERY
Baby Bennett Retractor

humerus

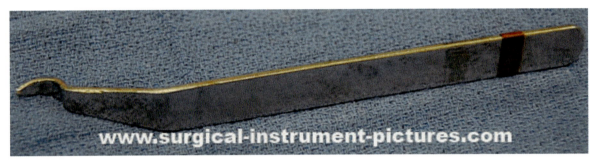

Surgical Instrument: Baby Bennett
Alias: None
Use: Elevation and retraction
Additional Info: Typically used on small bones in the foot or wrist

Beaver Blade Handle

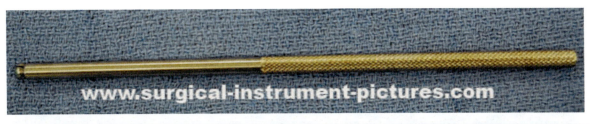

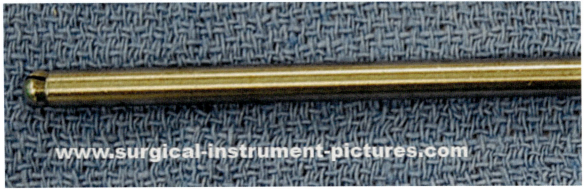

Surgical Instrument: Beaver Blade Handle
Alias: None
Use: Cutting
Additional Info: Typically for small orthopedic surgeries such as hand and foot surgery

Adson Bipolar Forceps

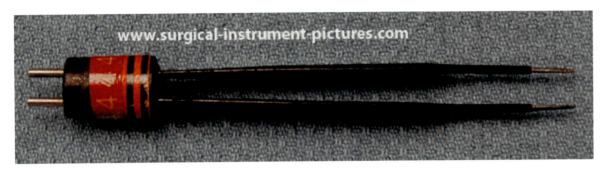

Surgical Instrument: Adson Bipolar Forceps
Alias: None
Use: Coagulation
Additional Info: For small orthopedic surgery, current is bipolar in nature so unlike a bovie it doesn't require a grounding pad and is often preferred around delicate vessels and nerves because it produces less thermal dispersion

Bone Tamp

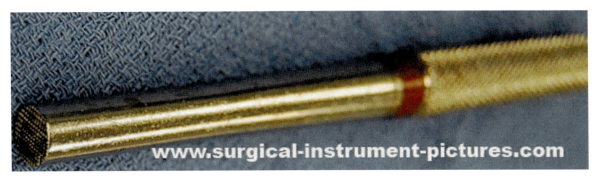

Surgical Instrument: Bone Tamp
Alias: None
Use: Compaction of bone
Additional Info: None

Brun Currette

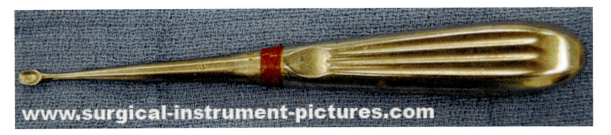

Surgical Instrument: Brun Currette
Alias: None
Use: Curretting bone
Additional Info: Available with many cup sizes and varying degrees of angle for the head

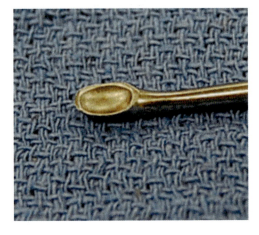

Cobb Elevator

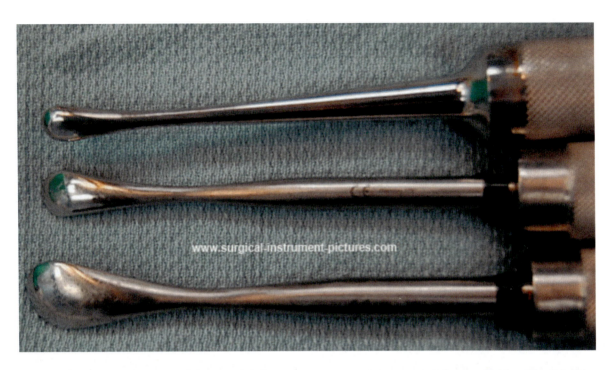

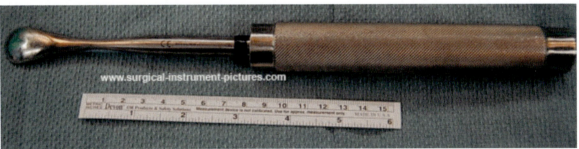

Surgical Instrument: Cobb elevator
Alias: None
Use: Elevating and blunt dissection
Additional Info: None

K-Wire Cutter

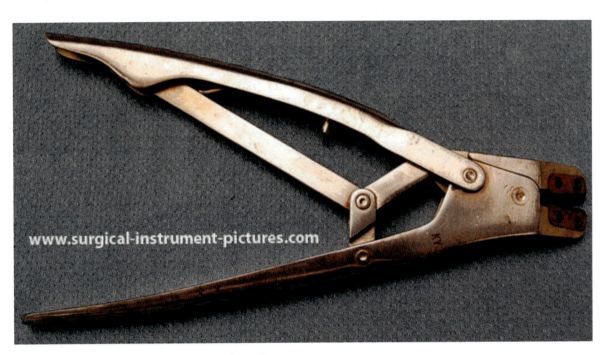

Surgical Instrument: K-Wire Cutter
Alias: Pin Cutter
Use: Cutting metal wire and K-Wires
Additional Info: None

Freer Elevator

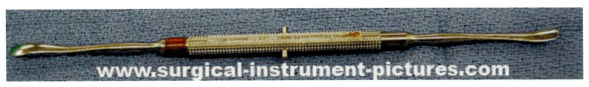

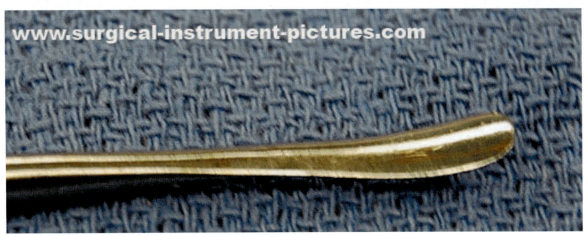

Surgical Instrument: Freer Elevator
Alias: None
Use: Elevating and blunt dissection
Additional Info: Typical in smaller orthopedic surgeries

Deep Gelpi

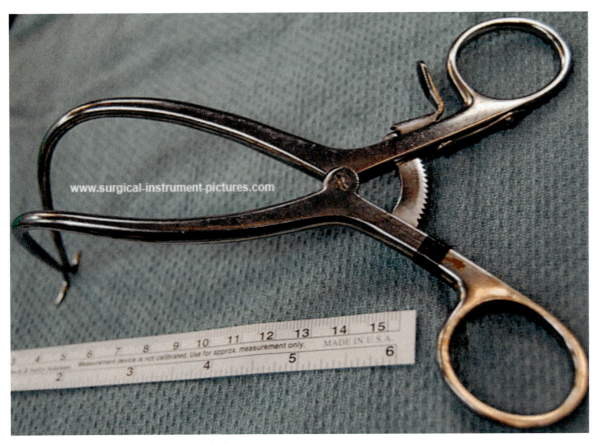

Surgical Instrument: Gelpi
Alias: None
Use: Retraction
Additional Info: Self-retaining retractor common in spine surgery

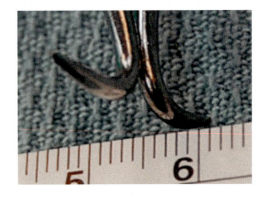

Ragnell Retractor

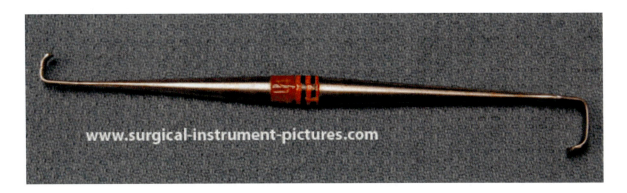

Surgical Instrument: Ragnell
Alias: None
Use: Retraction
Additional Info: Small orthopedic retractor

Hoen Elevator

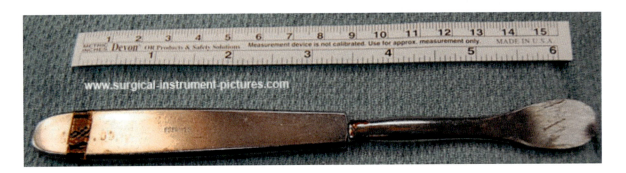

Surgical Instrument: Hoen Elevator
Alias: None
Use: Blunt dissection
Additional Info: None

Small & Large Key

~~Hoke Osteotome~~

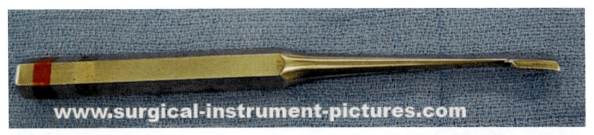

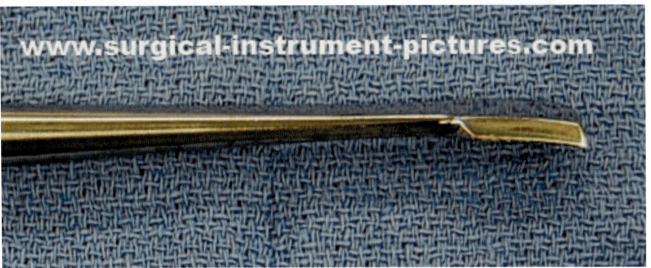

Surgical Instrument: Hoke Osteotome
Alias: None
Use: Dissection
Additional Info: None

Key Elevator

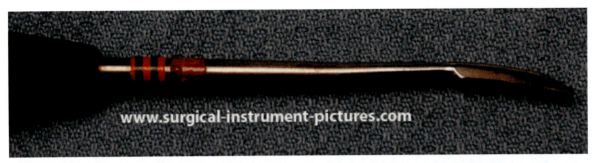

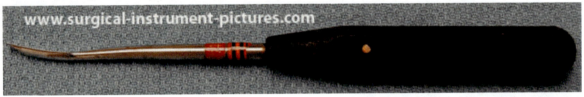

Surgical Instrument: Key Elevator
Alias: None
Use: Dissection
Additional Info: None

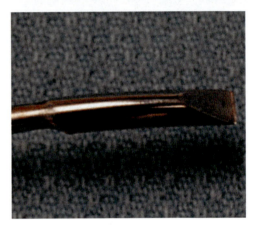

Kocher Clamp

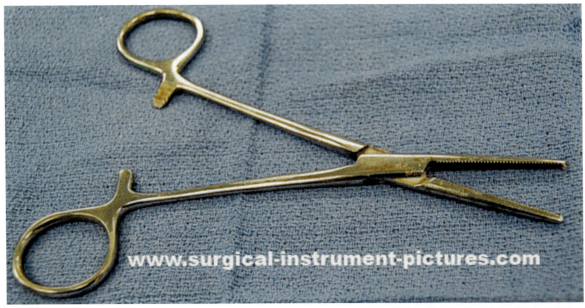

Surgical Instrument: Kocher Clamp
Alias: None
Use: Grasping
Additional Info: For grasping bone or fascia during general surgery.

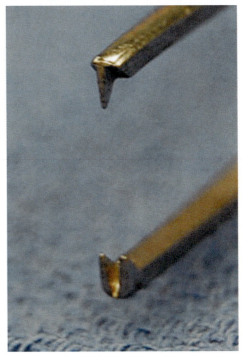

flat / straight / curve

Lambotte Osteotome

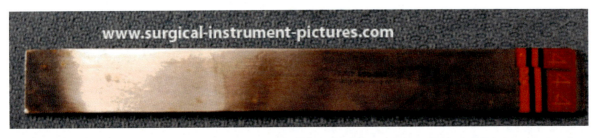

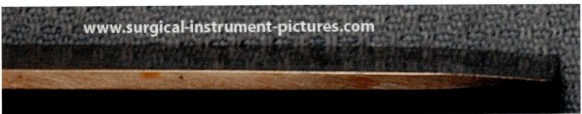

Surgical Instrument: Lambotte Osteotome
Alias: Lambot
Use: Dissection
Additional Info: Available both straight and curved at the tip. Often used to take hip and bone grafts

Putti Rasp

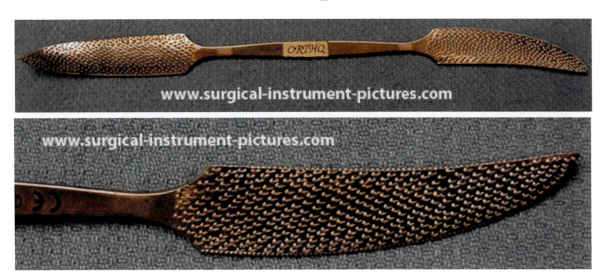

Surgical Instrument: Putti Rasp
Alias: None
Use: Grating
Additional Info: Rasping bone; often used to contour bone after amputations

Rainey Forceps

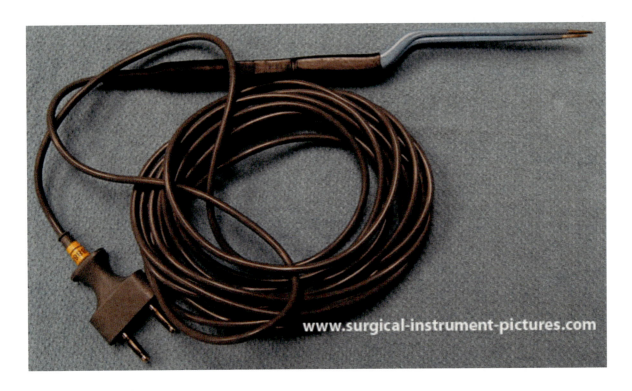

Surgical Instrument: Rainey Forceps
Alias: None
Use: Cautery
Additional Info: Confused with a bipolar, this has monopolar current and therefore requires a grounding pad

Rongeur

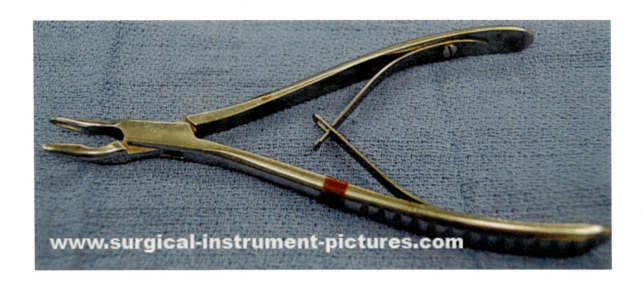

Surgical Instrument: Rongeur
Alias: None
Use: Cutting
Additional Info: None

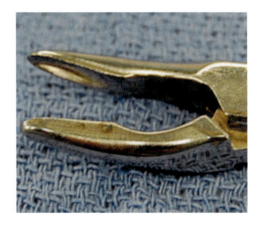

Double Action Rongeur

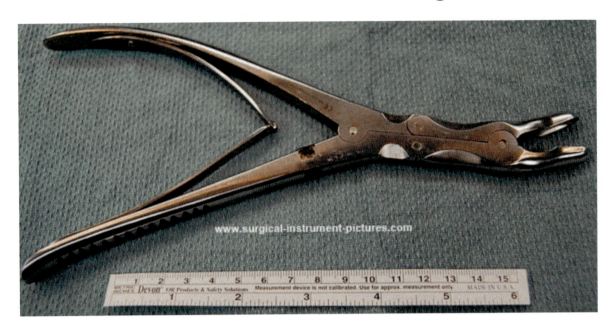

Surgical Instrument: Rongeur
Alias: None
Use: Cutting
Additional Info: Larger than a single action rongeur

finger retractors &

Sauerburch Retractor

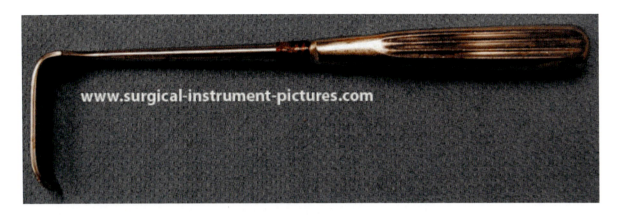

Surgical Instrument: Sauerburch Retractor
Alias: Sauer
Use: Retraction
Additional Info: Medium sized orthopedic retractor

Spring Self-Retaining Retractor

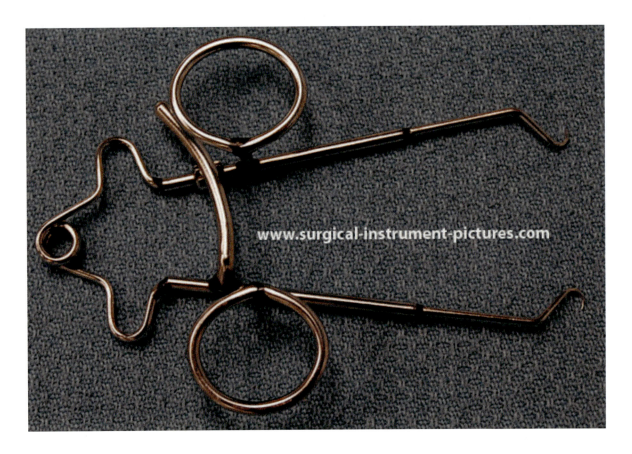

Surgical Instrument: Spring self-retaining retractor
Alias: None
Use: retraction
Additional Info: Small self-retaining retractor common for hand surgery

Tendon Passer

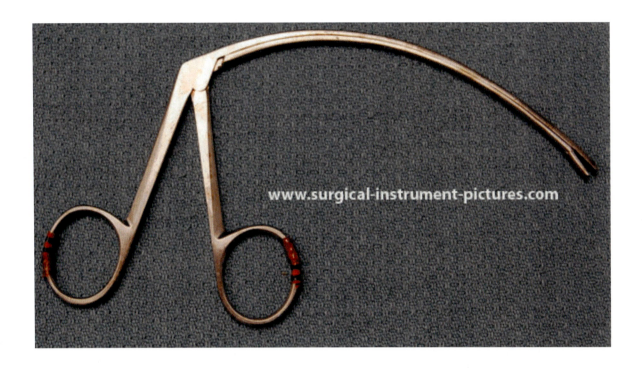

Surgical Instrument: Tendon Passer
Alias: None
Use: None
Additional Info: Used in hand and foot surgery for passing tendons for reattachment.

VASCULAR SURGERY

AP Suction Tip

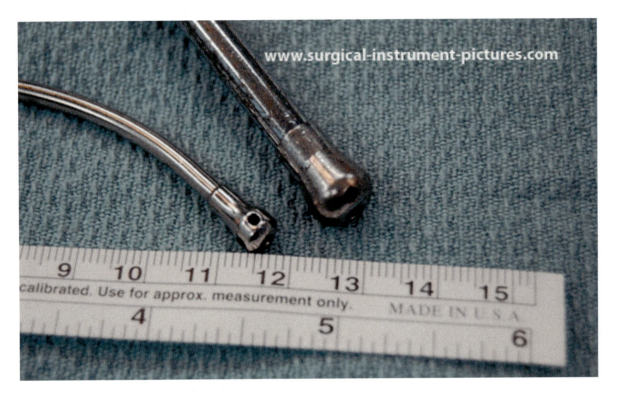

Surgical Instrument: AP Suction
Alias: Tonsil Suction
Use: Suction
Additional Info: Pictured to the left of the similar but larger yankauer suction tip

Alexander Periosteotome

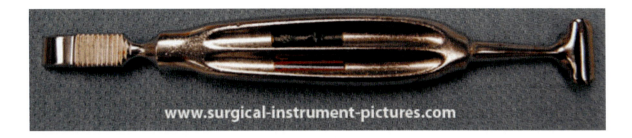

Surgical Instrument: Alexander Periosteotome
Alias: None
Use: Dissection
Additional Info: Typically found in chest vascular sets

Aortic Clamp

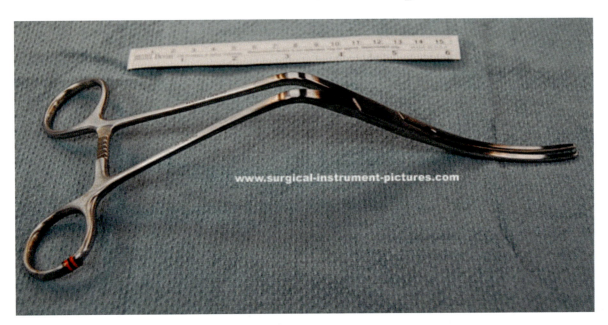

Surgical Instrument: Aortic Clamp
Alias: None
Use: Clamping
Additional Info: Non-Traumatic debakey like teeth used to clamp the Aorta in a AAA repair

Glover Clamp

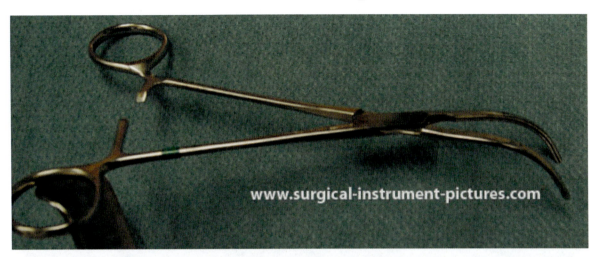

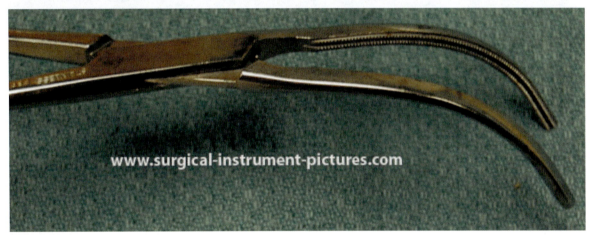

Surgical Instrument: Glover
Alias: None
Use: Clamping
Additional Info: Large non-traumatic vascular clamp

Burford Finochietto

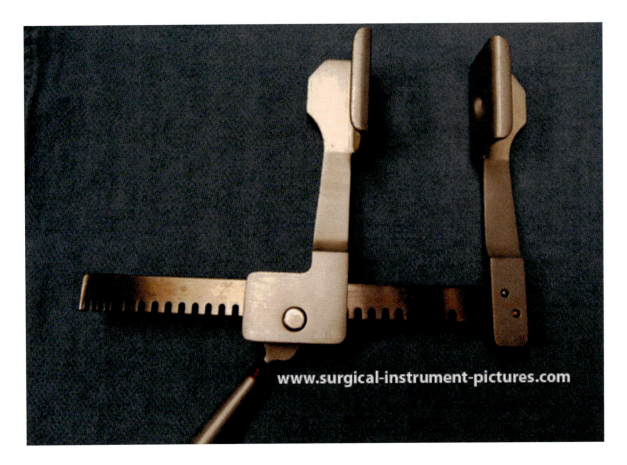

Surgical Instrument: Finochietto
Alias: None
Use: Retraction
Additional Info: Used to spread and retract the rib cage for thoracic surgery

Finochietto Blade

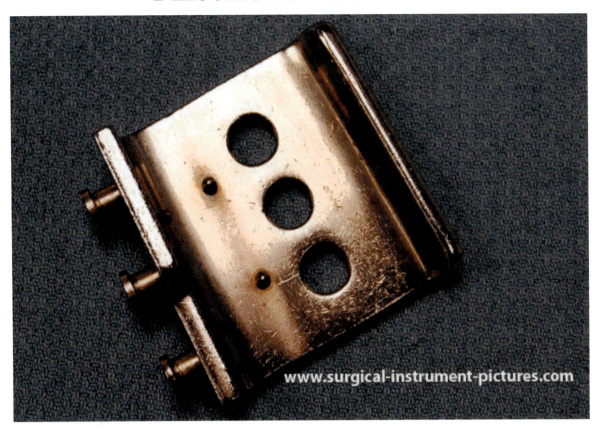

Surgical Instrument: Finochietto Blade
Alias: None
Use: Retraction
Additional Info: Variable in size, attached to a finochetti retractor

Javid Carotid Clamp

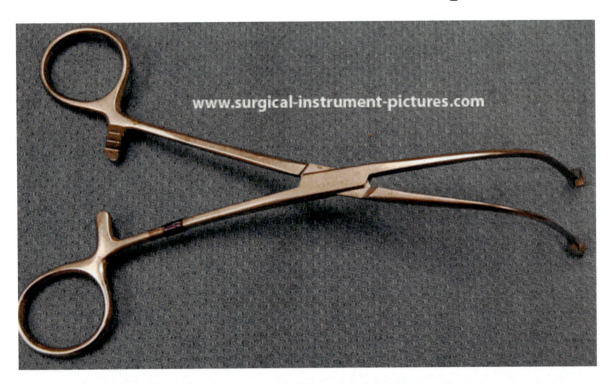

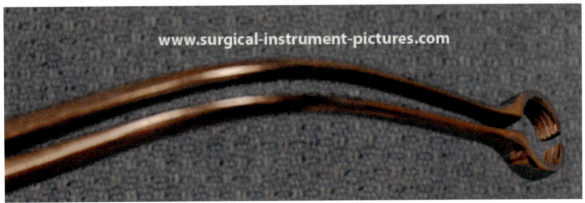

Surgical Instrument: Javid Carotid Clamp
Alias: None
Use: Clamping
Additional Info: For control of the carotic artery

Castro Viejo Needle Holder, Locking

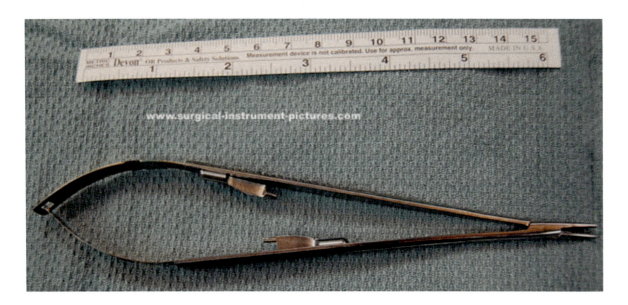

Surgical Instrument: Castro Viejo
Alias: None
Use: Suturing
Additional Info: Fine needle driver for small vessels and nerves available both locking and non-locking

Hemo Clip Applier

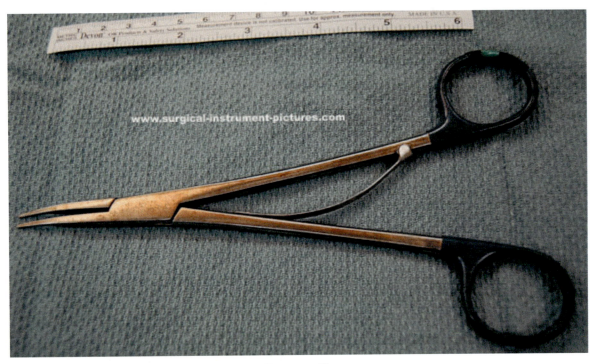

Surgical Instrument: Hemo Clip Applier
Alias: None
Use: Ligation
Additional Info: Used to ligate vessels available in both disposable and non-disposable varieties

Vein Retractor

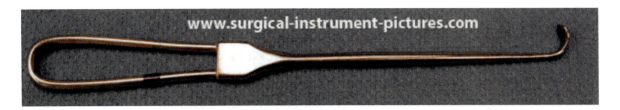

Surgical Instrument: Vein Retractor
Alias: None
Use: Vein retractor
Additional Info: None

Debakey Clamp

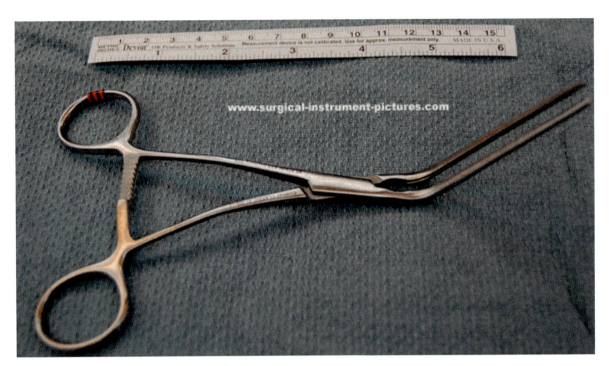

Surgical Instrument: Debakey Clamp
Alias: None
Use: Clamping large vessels
Additional Info: Multi-purpose non-traumatic vascular clamp. See the next page for a close up of the jaws

Debakey Clamp

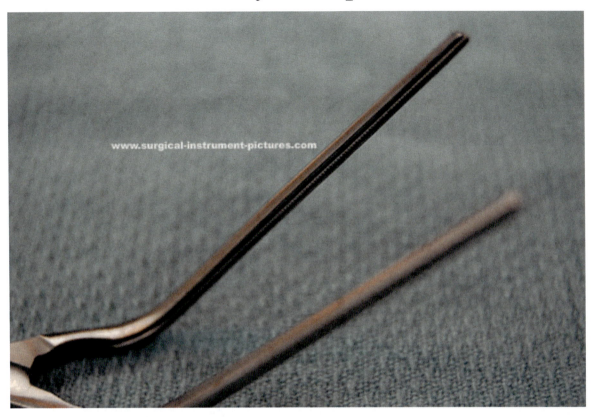

Surgical Instrument: Debakey Clamp
Additional Info: Multi purpose non-traumatic vascular clamp

Glover, Angled

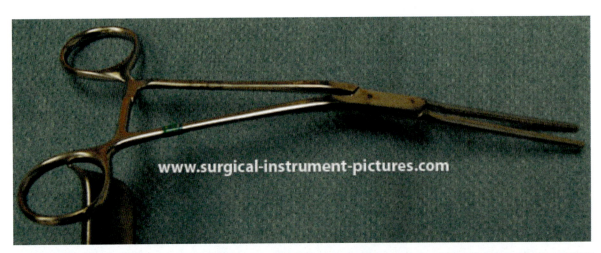

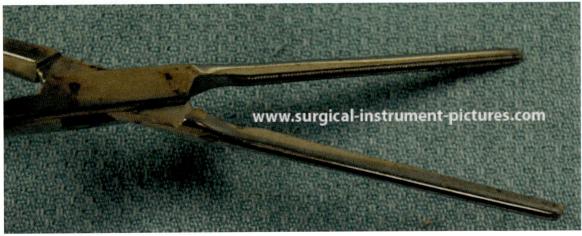

Surgical Instrument: Glover, Angled
Alias: None
Use: Clamping
Additional Info: Non-traumatic vascular clamp

Detrich Forceps

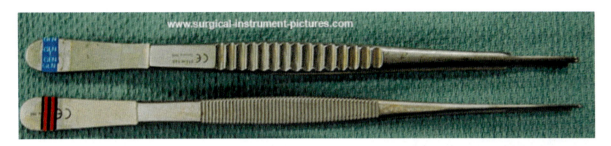

Surgical Instrument: Detrich Forceps
Alias: None
Use: Grasping
Additional Info: Smaller but similar to the debakey forceps above, detrich forceps are a fine vascular pickup

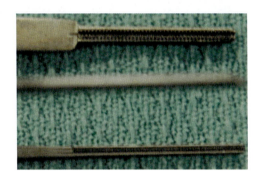

Doyan Rib Rasp

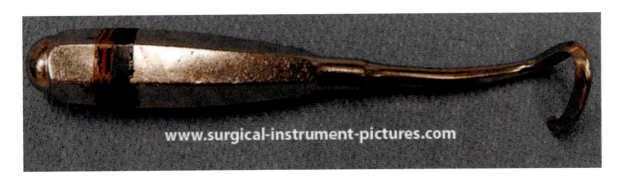

Surgical Instrument: Doyan
Alias: None
Use: Dissection
Additional Info: Common to the thoracic set

Scapula Retractor

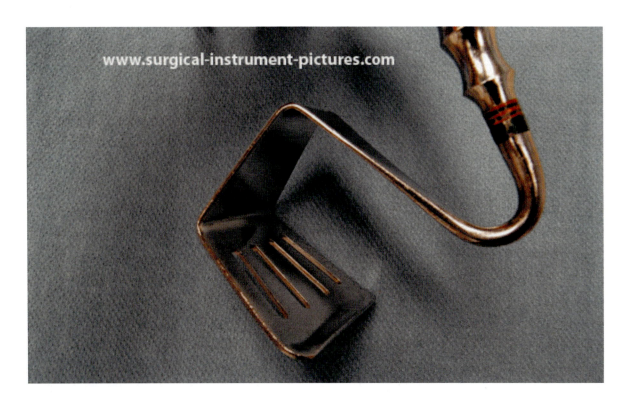

Surgical Instrument: Scapula Retractor
Alias: None
Use: Retraction
Additional Info: Common thoracic retractor

Karchner Internal Carotid Clamp

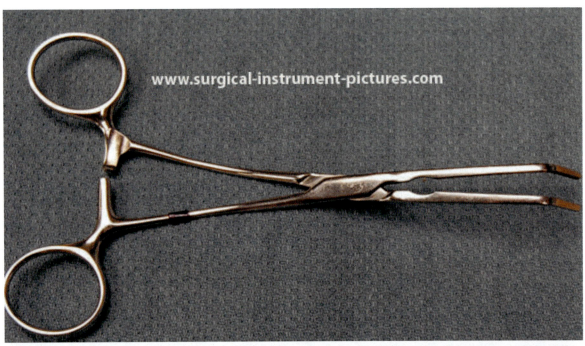

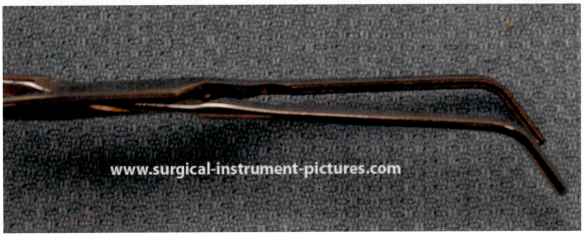

Surgical Instrument: Karchner Clamp
Alias: Internal Carotid
Use: Clamping the Carotid Artery
Additional Info: Exclusive to carotid surgery

Wylie External Carotid Clamp

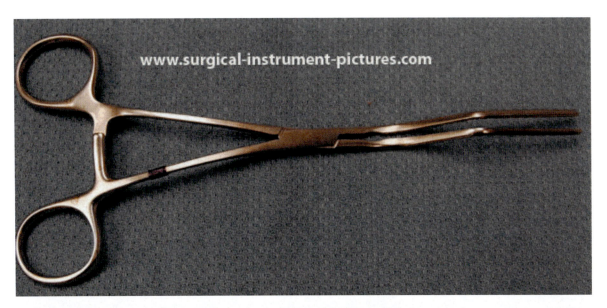

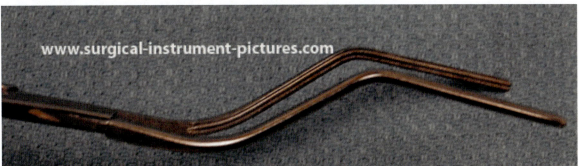

Surgical Instrument: Wylie External Carotid Clamp
Alias: None
Use: Clamping the external carotid artery
Additional Info: Exclusive to carotid surgery

Duval Lung Clamp

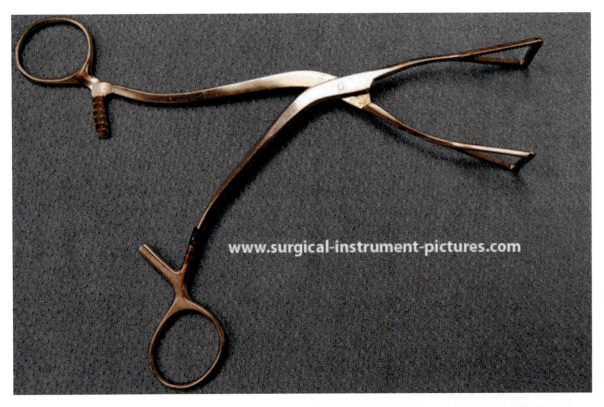

Surgical Instrument: Duval Lung Clamp
Alias: None
Use: Grasping
Additional Info: For grasping the lung

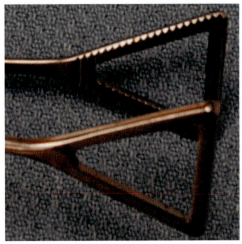

Fogarty Clamp

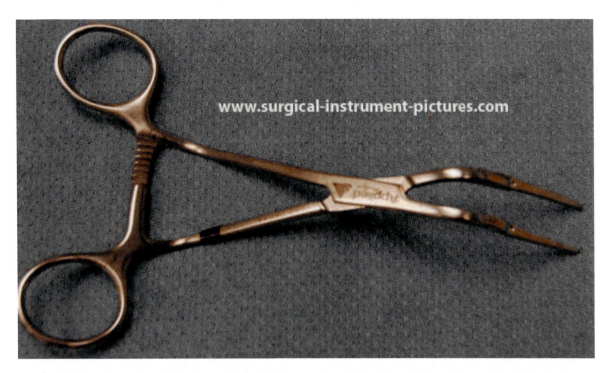

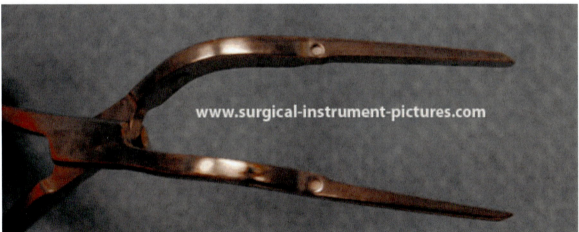

Surgical Instrument: Fogarty Clamp
Alias: None
Use: Clamping
Additional Info: Plastic forgarty attachments are required for the jaws of the clamp

Gerald Forceps

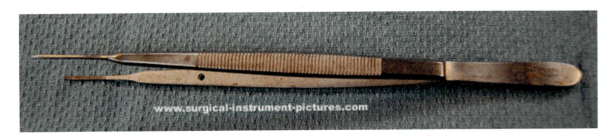

Surgical Instrument: Gerald Forceps
Alias: None
Use: Grasping
Additional Info: Small vascular pickup

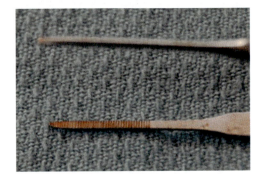

Glover Clamp, Straight

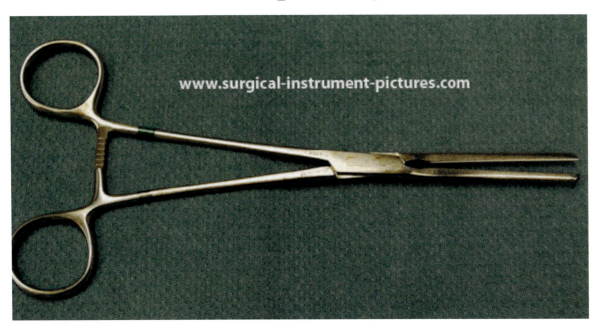

Surgical Instrument: Glover, Straight
Alias: None
Use: Clamping
Additional Info: Non-traumatic large vascular clamp

Henley Retractor

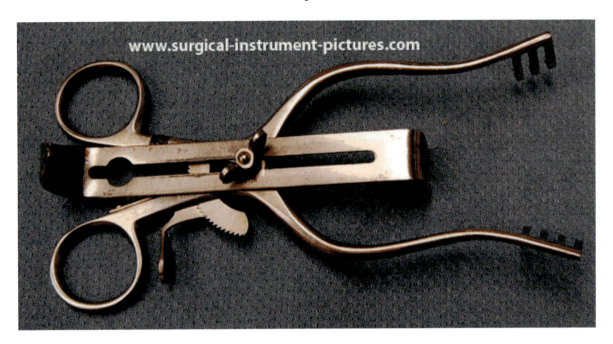

Surgical Instrument: Henley Retractor
Alias: None
Use: Retraction
Additional Info: Similar to a weitlaner with the addition of a vertical retraction blade

Jake Clamp

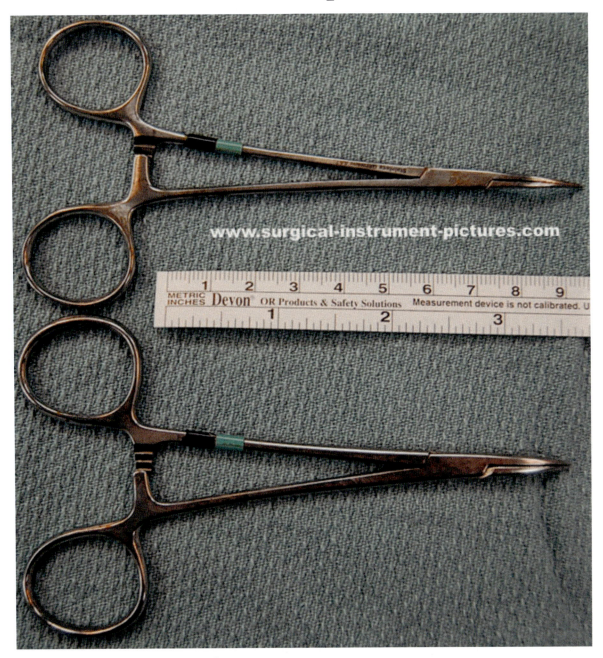

Surgical Instrument: Jake
Alias: None
Use: Fine dissection, clamping
Additional Info: Pictured above the mosquito clamp, notice the smaller jaw of the jake

Statinsky Clamp

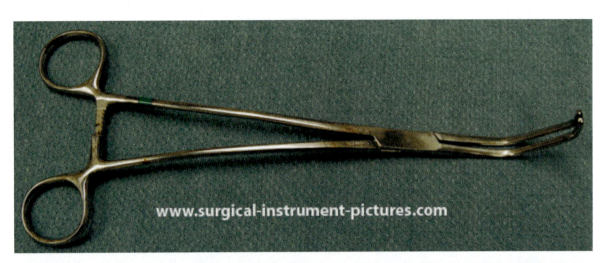

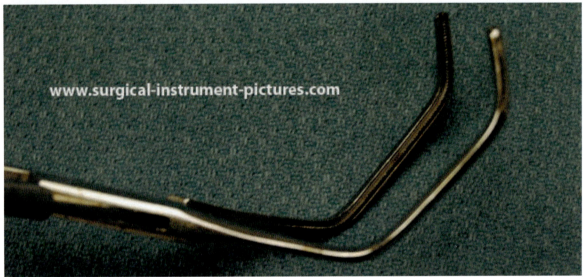

Surgical Instrument: Statinsky
Alias: None
Use: Clamping
Additional Info: Large vascular clamp

Potts Scissors

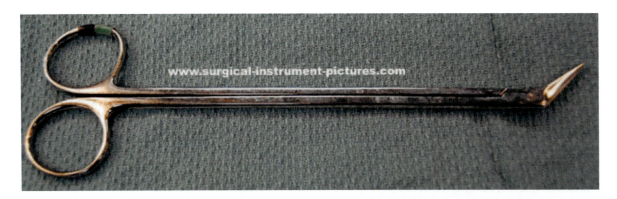

Surgical Instrument: Potts Scissors
Alias: None
Use: Cutting
Additional Info: Used for cutting down the shaft of the vessel in preparation for a graft

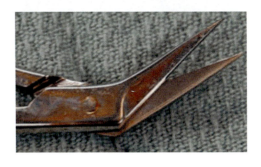

Rib Approximator

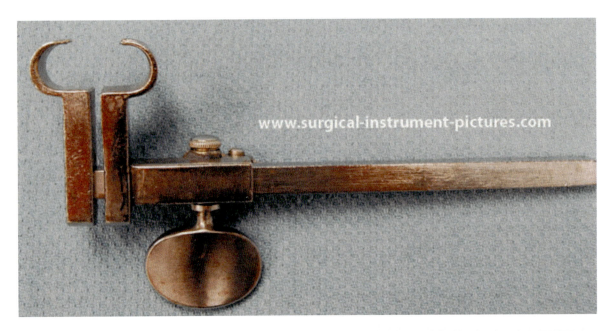

Surgical Instrument: Rib Approximator
Alias: None
Use: Bringing the ribs together
Additional Info: Common to the thoracic set

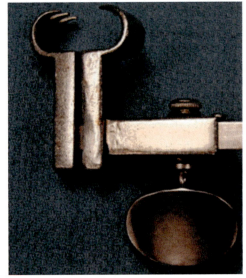

Bethune Rib Shears

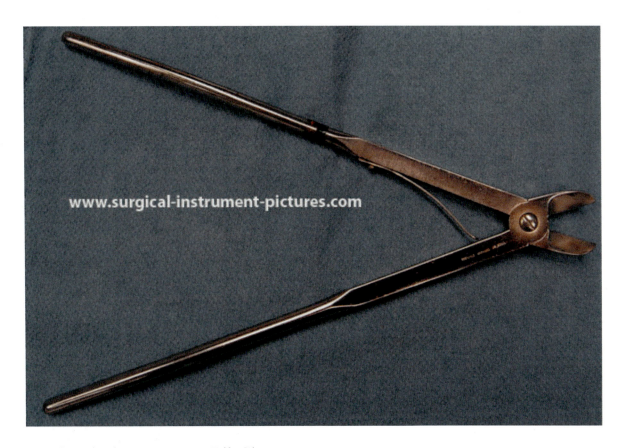

Surgical Instrument: Rib Shear
Alias: None
Use: Cutting
Additional Info: Large bone cutting shear

Rummel Stylet

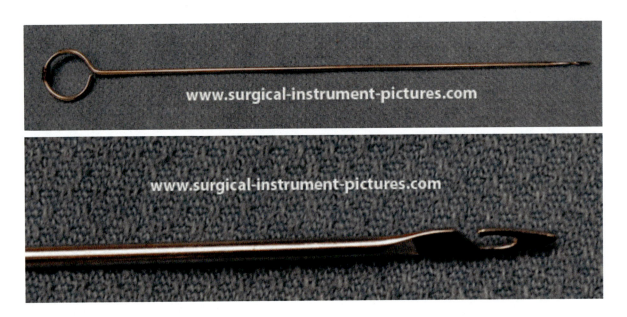

Surgical Instrument: Rummel Stylet
Alias: None
Additional Info: Commonly found in vascualar instrument sets

Statinsky Scissors

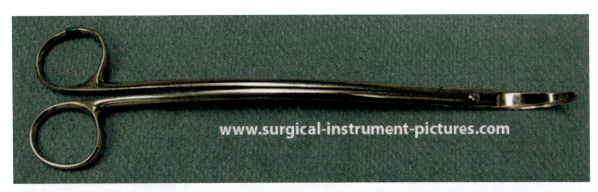

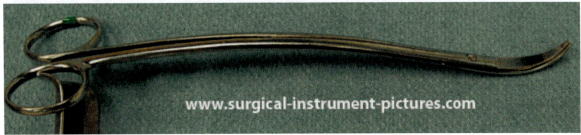

Surgical Instrument: Statinsky Scissors
Alias: None
Use: Cutting
Additional Info: Large chest vascular scissors

Sauerbruch Rongeur

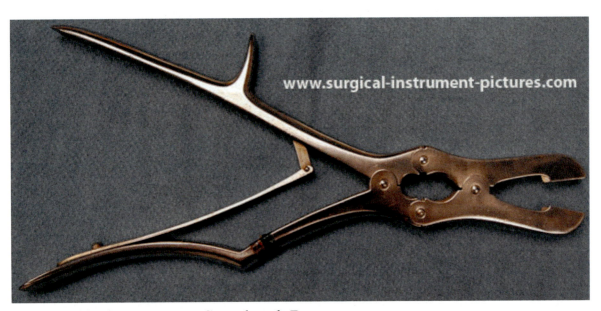

Surgical Instrument: Sauerbruch Rongeur
Alias: Box Cutter
Use: Cutting
Additional Info: Large double action rongeur found in the chest vascular set

Vessel Irrigator

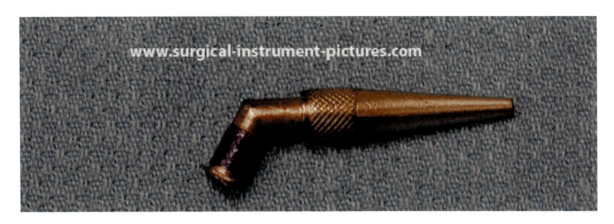

Surgical Instrument: Vessel Irrigator
Alias: None
Use: Irrigation
Additional Info: Used for irrigation of blood vessels usually with heparinized saline

Vessel Probe

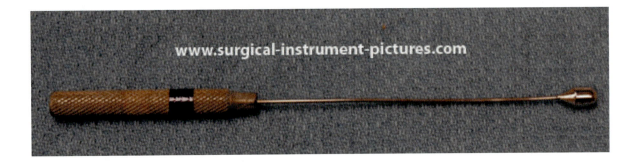

Surgical Instrument: Vessel probe
Alias: None
Use: Probe
Additional Info: Used to assess the internal diameter and any blockages within blood vessels, typically between 1-6mm in diameter

Neuro-Spine Surgery

90 Degree Dural Elevator

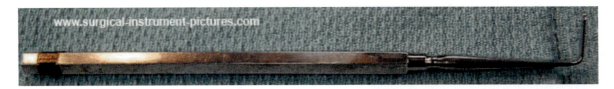

Surgical Instrument: 90 Degree Dural Elevator
Alias: Hockey Stick
Use: Dissection

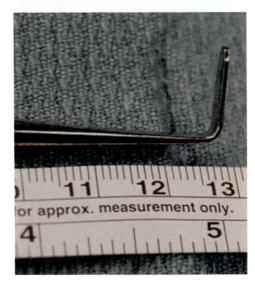

Bayonette Bipolar Forceps

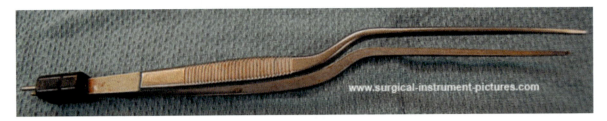

Surgical Instrument: Bayonette Bipolar
Alias: None
Use: Coagulation
Additional Info: Can also have an irrigation tip not pictured here for neurosurgery

Bayonette Forceps

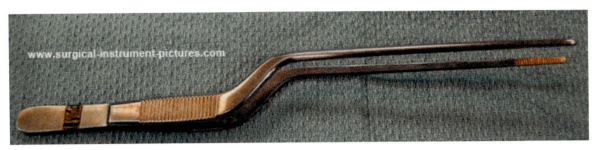

Surgical Instrument: Bayonette Forceps
Use: Grasping
Additional Info: Common to both ENT and Neurosurgery

Cherry Scissors

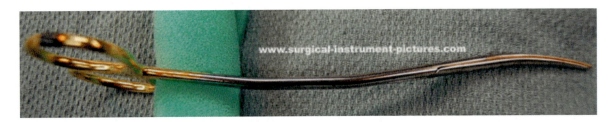

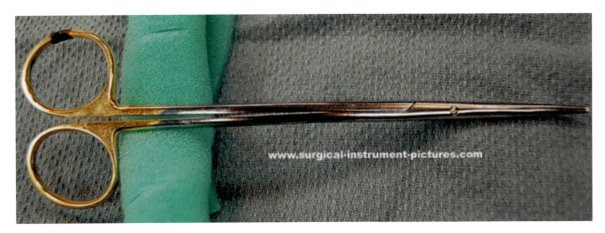

Surgical Instrument: Cherry Scissors
Alias: None
Use: Cutting
Additional Info: Common to neuro surgery

Cushing Forceps w/ teeth

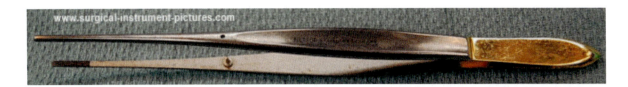

Surgical Instrument: Cushing forceps
Alias: None
Use: Grasping
Additional Info: Common pickups for use in craniotomies

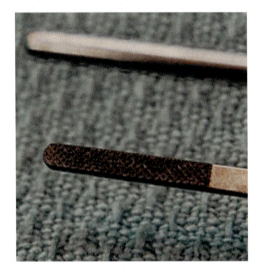

Gelpi Deep

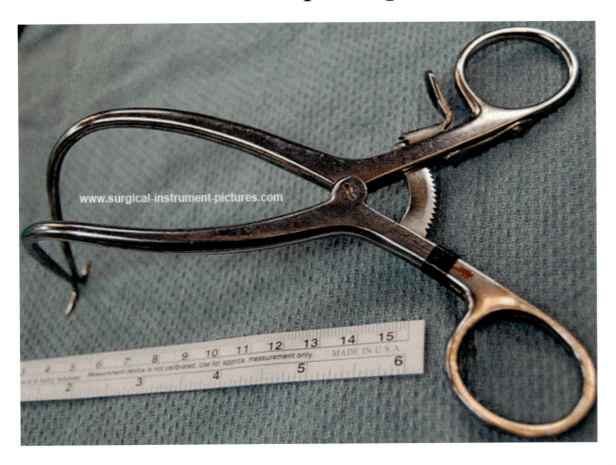

Surgical Instrument: Deep Gelpi
Alias: None
Use: Retraction
Additional Info: Common for retraction during spine surgery

Gelpi, Shallow

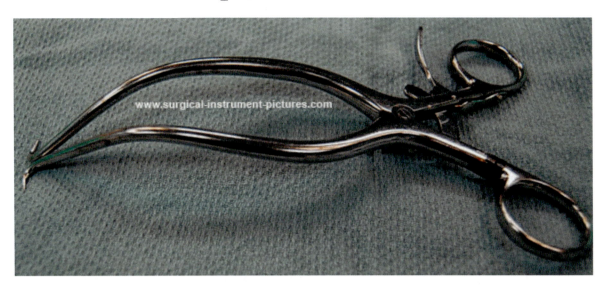

Surgical Instrument: Shallow Gelpi
Alias: None
Use: Retraction
Additional Info: None

Kerrison Ronguer

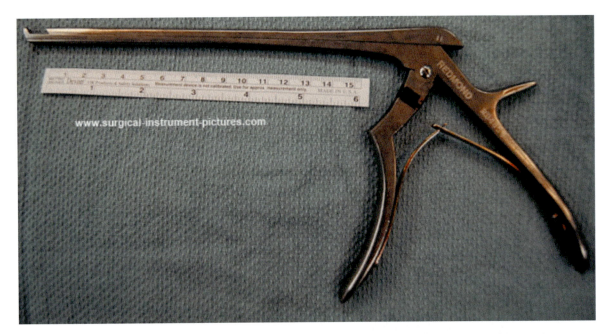

Surgical Instrument: Kerrison Ronguer
Alias: Kerrison Punch
Use: Cutting bone
Additional Info: For cutting bone in spine and cranial surgery

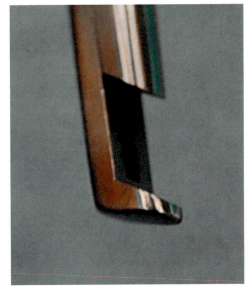

Nerve Hook

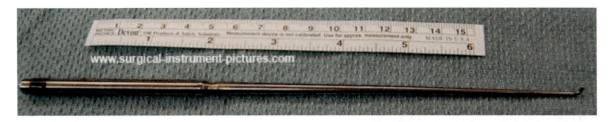

Surgical Instrument: Nerve Hook
Alias: None
Use: Retraction
Additional Info: For retraction of small delicate neurological structures

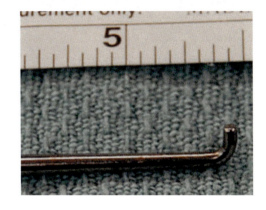

Dural Retractor

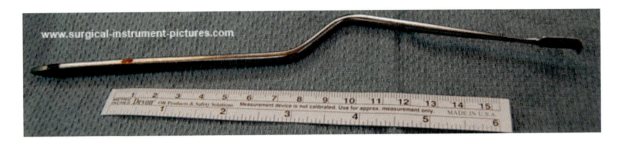

Surgical Instrument: Dural Retractor
Alias: None
Use: Retraction
Additional Info: Exclusive to spine surgery

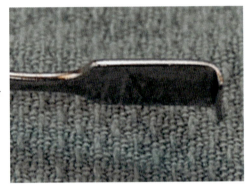

Penfield 1

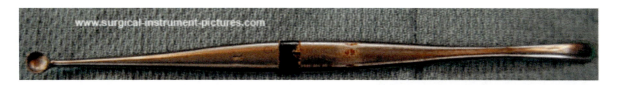

Surgical Instrument: Penfield 1
Alias: None
Use: Dissection
Additional Info: None

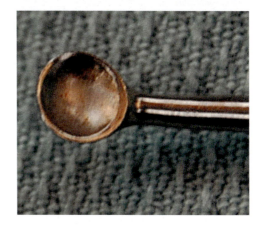

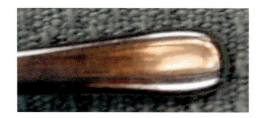

Penfield 2

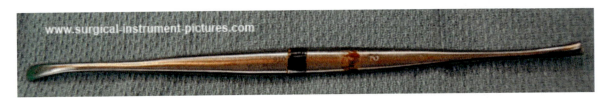

Surgical Instrument: Penfield 2
Alias: None
Use: Dissection
Additional Info: None

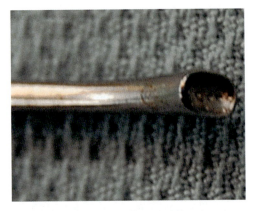

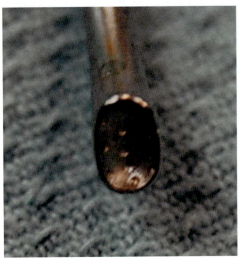

Penfield 3

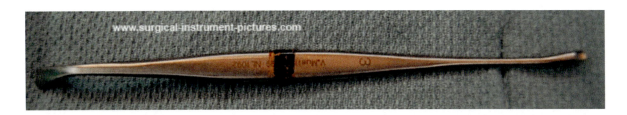

Surgical Instrument: Penfield 3
Alias: None
Use: Dissection
Additional Info: None

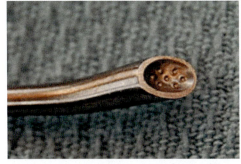

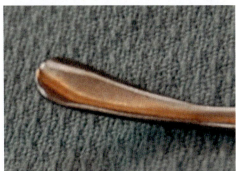

Penfield 4

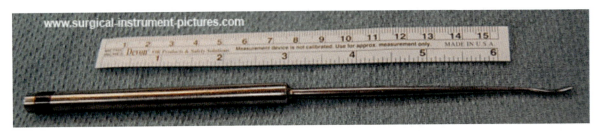

Surgical Instrument: Penfield 4
Alias: None
Use: Dissection
Additional Info: Often bone wax will be applied to the back side of the Penfield 4

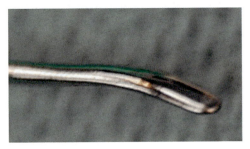

Penfields 1-4

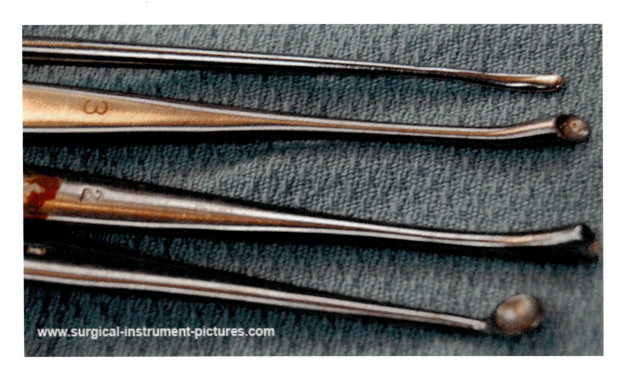

Surgical Instrument: Penfield 1-4
Alias: None
Use: Dissection
Additional Info: From Penfield 1-4 side by side

Pituitary Forceps

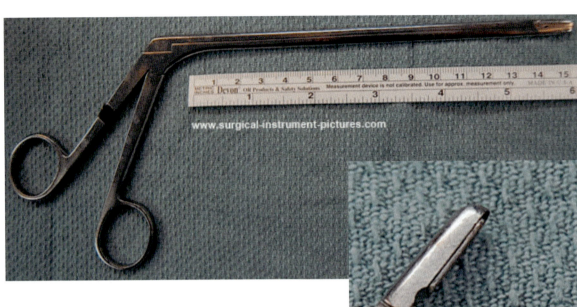

Surgical Instrument: Pituitary Forceps
Alias: None
Use: Grasping
Additional Info: Available in different angles. Pictured to the side are the straight and up biting types

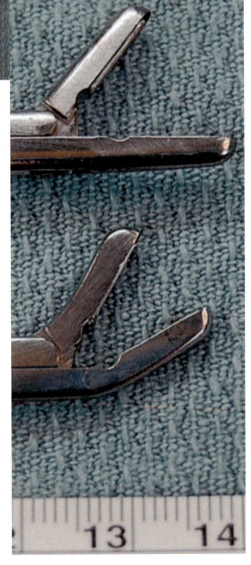

Curve/Angle Wheatlander

Cerebellar Retractor

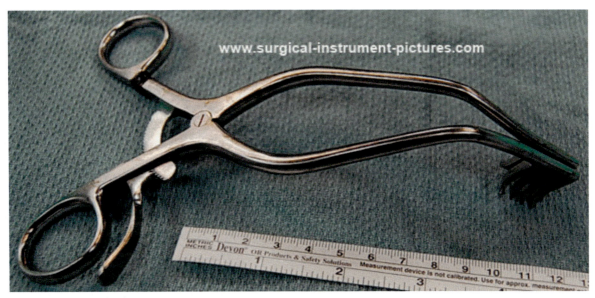

Surgical Instrument: Cerebellar Retractor
Alias: None
Use: Retraction
Additional Info: Retraction for cranial and cervical procedures

Woodson Elevator

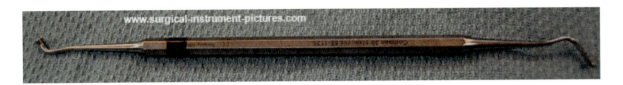

Surgical Instrument: Woodson
Alias: Dental
Use: Elevator/Dissector
Additional Info: Typical neurosurgical instrument

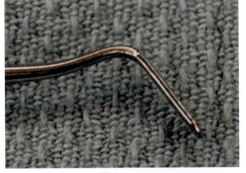

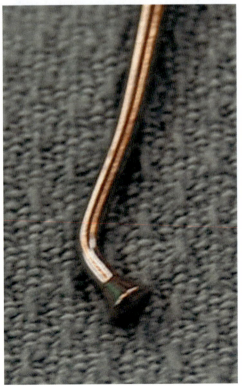

OB GYN Surgery

Tenaculum, Double Tooth

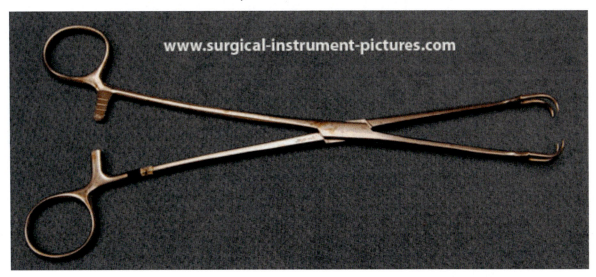

Surgical Instrument: Double Tooth Tenaculum
Alias: None
Use: Grasping
Additional Info: None

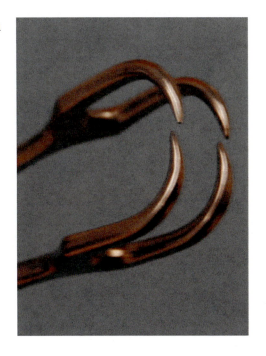

Weighted Vaginal Speculum

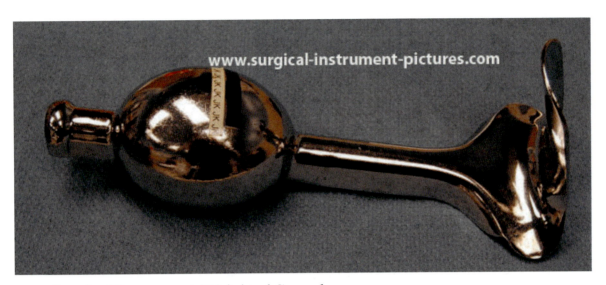

Surgical Instrument: Weighted Speculum
Alias: None
Use: Retraction
Additional Info: To provide exposure during vaginal procedures

Sims Retractor

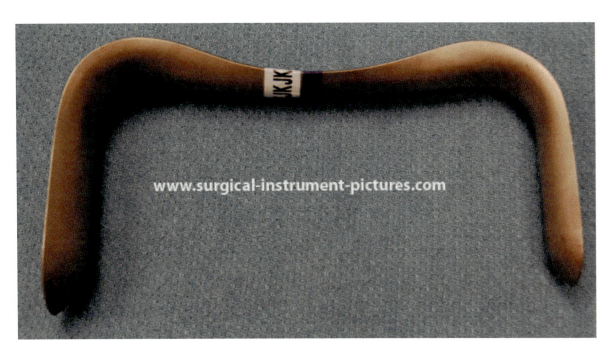

Surgical Instrument: Sims Retractor
Alias: None
Use: Retraction
Additional Info: To provide exposure during vaginal procedures

New York Speculum

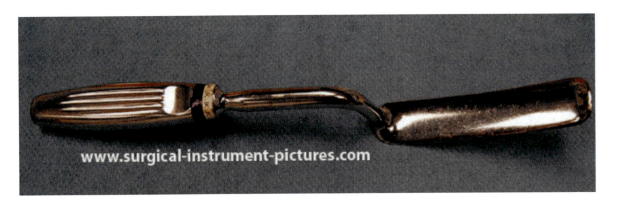

Surgical Instrument: New York Speculum
Alias: None
Use: Retraction
Additional Info: To provide exposure during vaginal procedures

Heaney-Simon Retractor

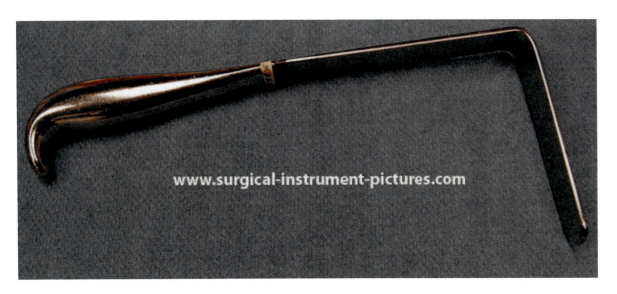

Surgical Instrument: Heaney-Simon
Alias: Heaney
Use: Retraction
Additional Info: To provide exposure during vaginal procedures

Jorgenson Scissors

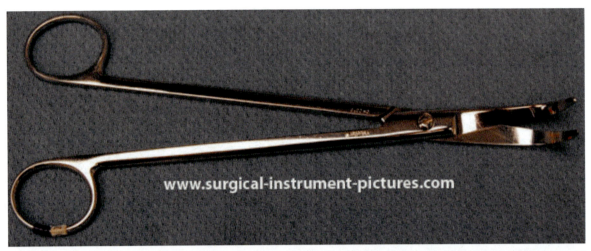

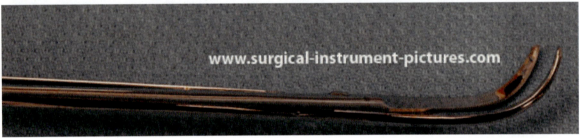

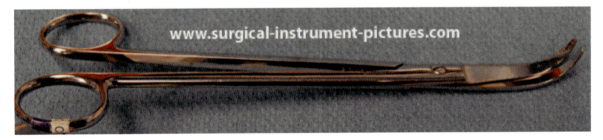

Surgical Instrument: Jorgenson Scissors
Alias: None
Use: Cutting
Additional Info: Curved GYN scissors commonly used during hysterectomies

Goelet Retractor

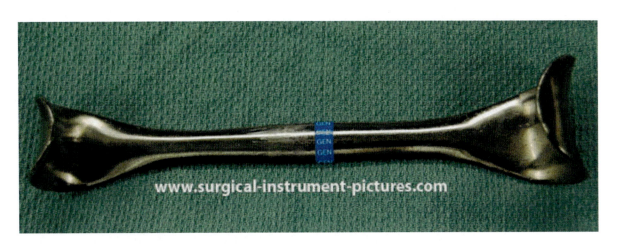

Surgical Instrument: Goelet
Alias: None
Use: Retraction
Additional Info: Abdominal retractor

Heaney-Ballantine Clamp, Straight

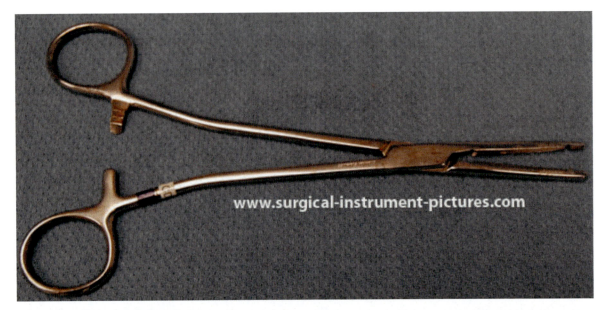

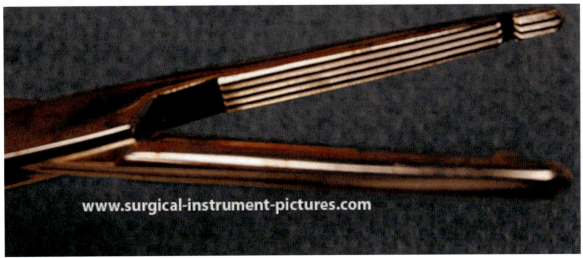

Surgical Instrument: Heany-Ballantine Clamp
Alias: Heany
Use: Clamping
Additional Info: Clamping of the uterus

Heany-Ballantine Clamp, Curved

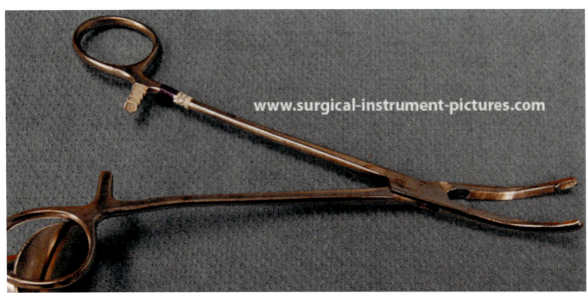

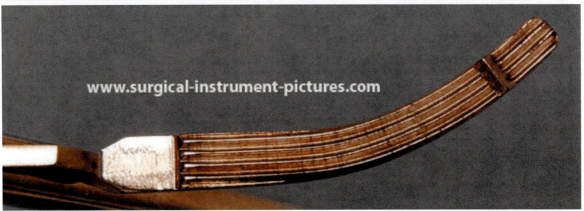

Surgical Instrument: Heany-Ballantine Clamp
Alias: Heany
Use: Clamping
Additional Info: Clamping of the uterus

Heaney Needle Holder

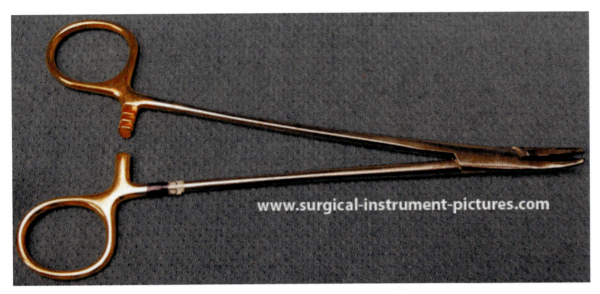

Surgical Instrument: Heaney Needle Holder
Alias: None
Use: Suturing
Additional Info: Recognized by the curved jaw

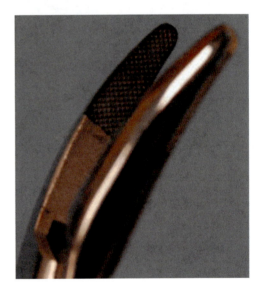

Jacob Tenaculum

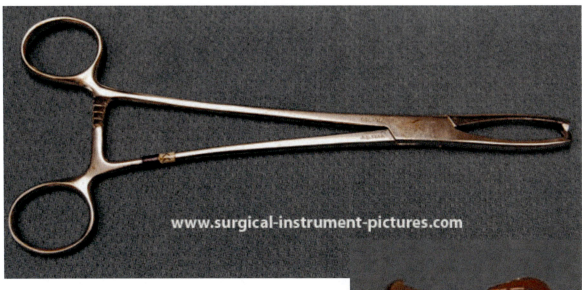

Surgical Instrument: Jacob Tenaculum
Alias: None
Use: Grasping
Additional Info: Common GYN grasping clamp

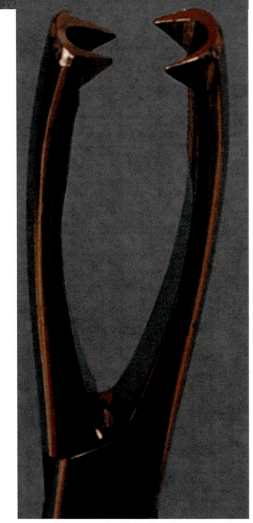

Lahey Clamp

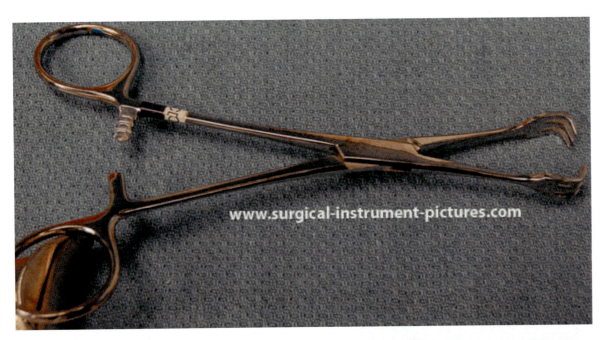

Surgical Instrument: Lahey
Alias: None
Use: Grasping
Additional Info: Common traumatic GYN grasping forcep

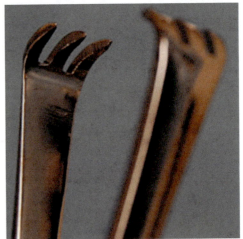

T Clamp

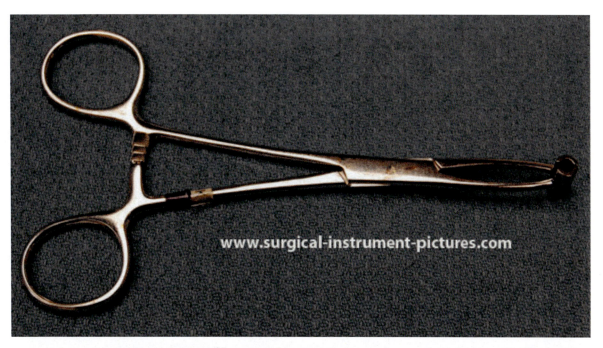

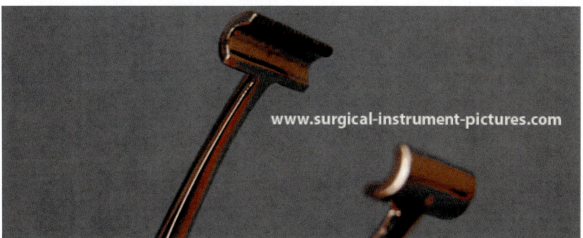

Surgical Instrument: T Clamp
Alias: None
Use: Clamping
Additional Info: Common non-traumatic GYN clamp

Balfour Retractor

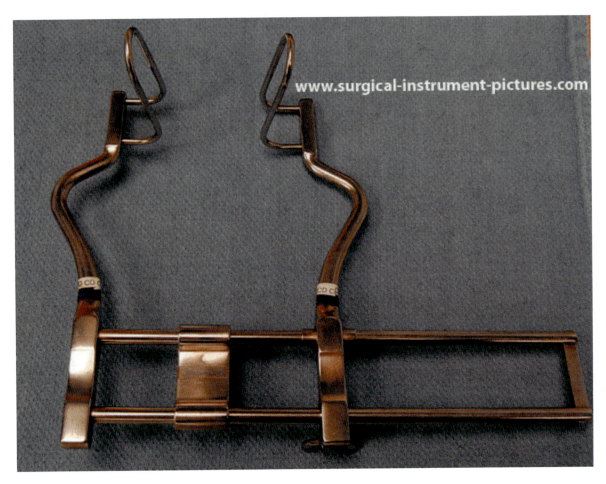

Surgical Instrument: Balfour
Alias: None
Use: Retraction
Additional Info: Common GYN and general surgical mid-sized abdominal retractor

Uterine Sound

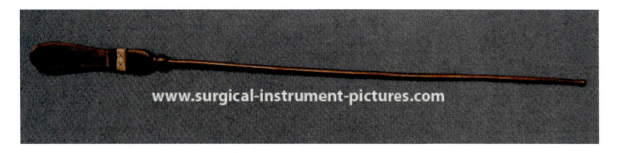

Surgical Instrument: Uterine Sound
Alias: None
Use: Probing
Additional Info: For probing the uterine cavity

Plastic and Cosmetic Surgery
Alm Retractor

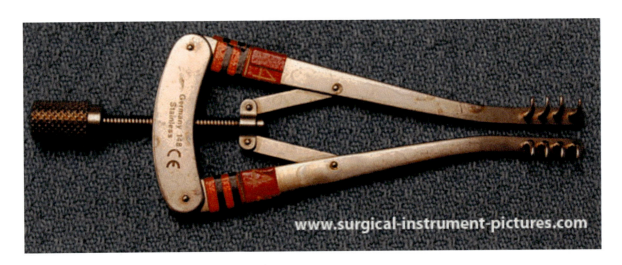

Surgical Instrument: Alm Retractor
Alias: None
Use: Retraction
Additional Info: Very small self-retaining retractor

Bishop Harmon Forceps

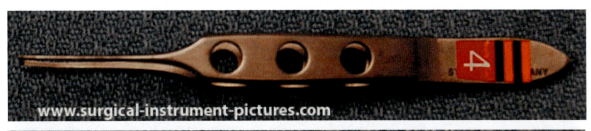

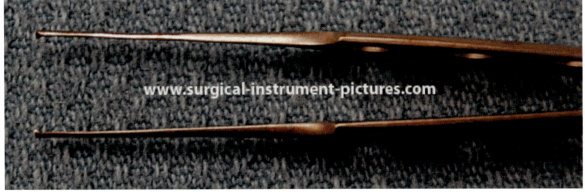

Surgical Instrument: Bishop Harmon Forceps
Alias: Bishops
Use: Grasping
Additional Info: Commonly for used for suturing in delicate cosmetic procedures

Hagar Scissors/Needle Holder

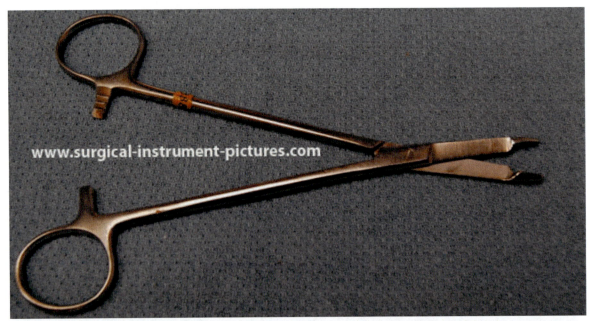

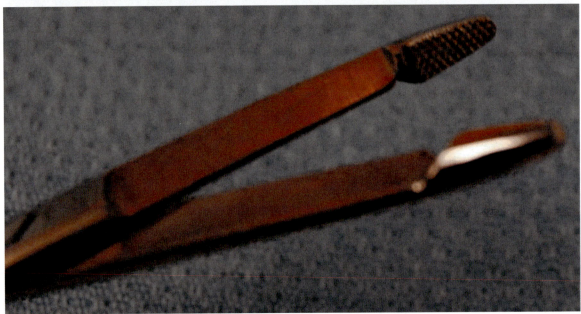

Surgical Instrument: Hagar Scissors.Needle Holder
Alias: None
Use: Cutting/suturing
Additional Info: Used to suture then cut the thread without changing instruments

Breast Template

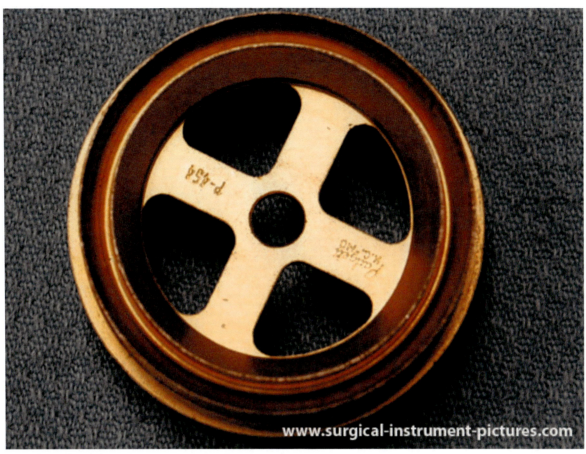

Surgical Instrument: Breast Template
Alias: Cookie Cutter
Use: Template
Additional Info: Used for the reconstruction of nipples durring breast surgery

Caliper

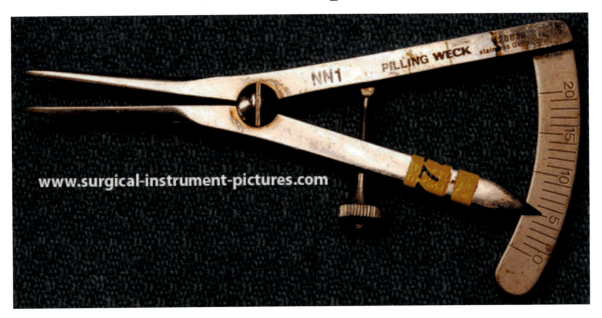

Surgical Instrument: Caliper
Alias: None
Use: Measurement
Additional Info: For ensuring symmetry in cosmetic surgery

Westcott Scissors

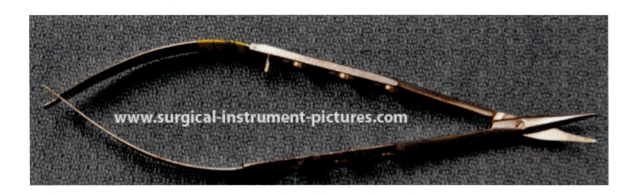

Surgical Instrument: Westcott Scissors
Alias: None
Use: Cutting
Additional Info: Delicate scissors for facial cosmetic surgery

Corneal Shield

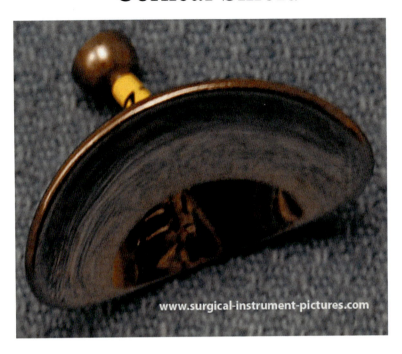

Surgical Instrument: Corneal Shield
Alias: None
Use: Eye Protection
Additional Info: Used to protect the eyes during facial plastic surgery and always used with an eye lubricant such as lacrilube to prevent corneal abrasions

Demar Retractor

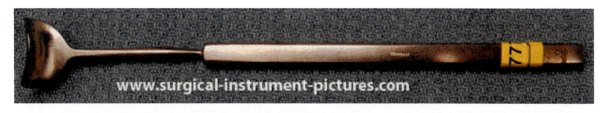

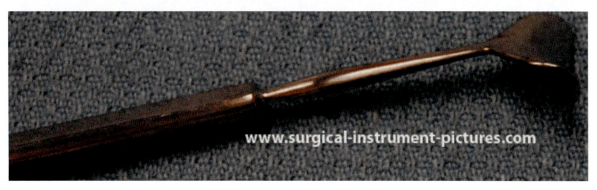

Surgical Instrument: Demar Retractor
Alias: None
Use: Retraction
Additional Info: Eye retractor for facial cosmetic surgery

Littler Scissors

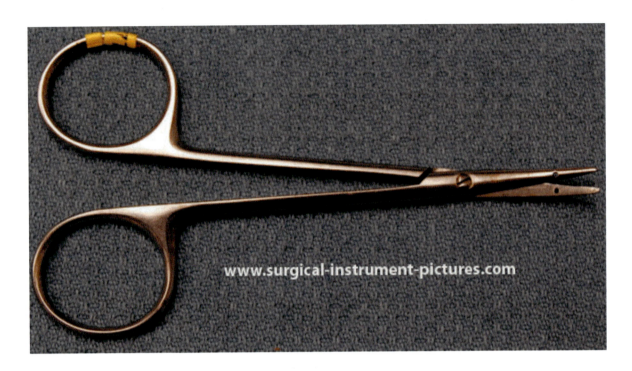

Surgical Instrument: Littler Scissors
Alias: None
Use: Cutting
Additional Info: Small tissue scissors for suture passing

Liposuction Cannula

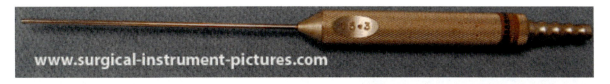

Surgical Instrument: Liposuction cannula
Alias: Lipo Cannula
Use: Hydro dissection
Additional Info: Used to cut and suction fat tissue during lipo suction

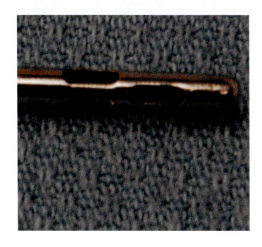

Klein Needle

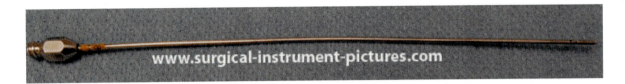

Surgical Instrument: Klein Needle
Alias: None
Use: Injection
Additional Info: Placed lipo fluid into the tissue to prepare the tissue for lipo suction

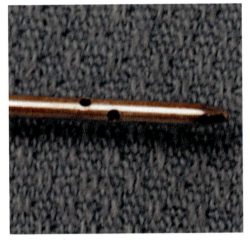

Fiber Optic Breast Retractor

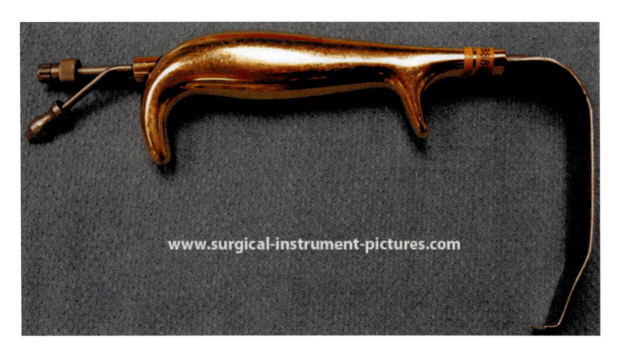

Surgical Instrument: Fiber Optic Breast Retractor
Alias: None
Use: Retraction
Additional Info: Used to see inside the cavity when placing breast implants

Fiber Optic Cord

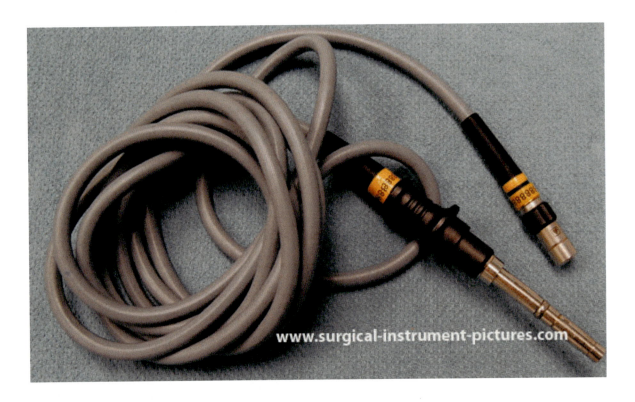

Surgical Instrument: Fiber Optic Cord
Alias: None
Use: Light Carrier
Additional Info: Multi-purpose light source

Freeman Retractor

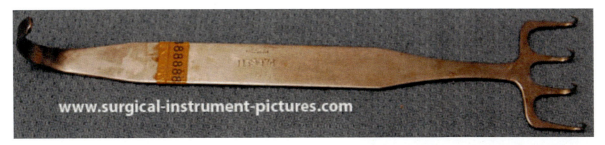

Surgical Instrument:
Alias: Facelift Retractor, Cat Paw
Use: Retraction
Additional Info: Common hand held retractor used in cosmetic surgery

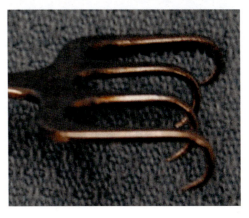

Facelift Scissors

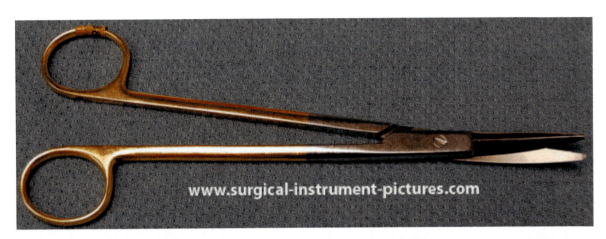

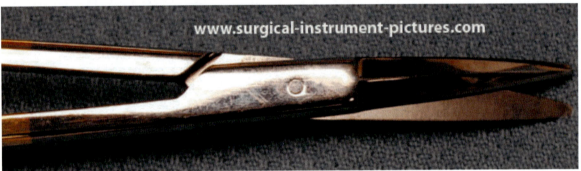

Surgical Instrument: Facelift Scissors
Alias: None
Use: Cutting
Additional Info: Used for cutting tissue in cosmetic surgical procedures, not limited to facelifts

Four Pronged Skin Hooks

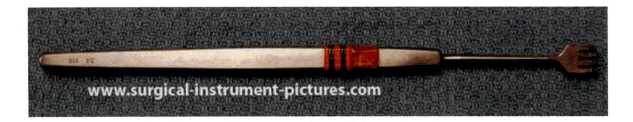

Surgical Instrument: Four Pronged Skin Hook
Alias: None
Use: Retraction
Additional Info: Small Skin Retractor

Gaurded Osteotome

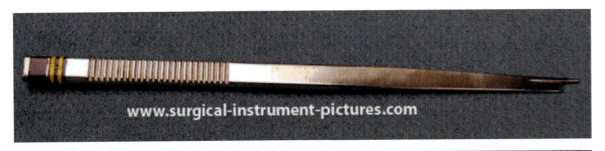

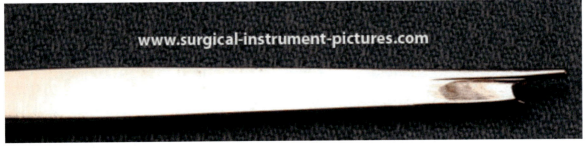

Surgical Instrument: Guarded Osteotome
Alias: None
Use: Cutting
Additional Info: Used for cutting septal and nasal bone during a rhinoplasty

Two Pronged Skin Hooks

Double skin hooks wider than Guthrie

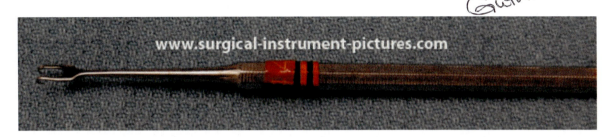

Surgical Instrument: Two Pronged Skin Hook
Alias: None
Use: Retraction
Additional Info: Small skin retractor

Iris Scissors

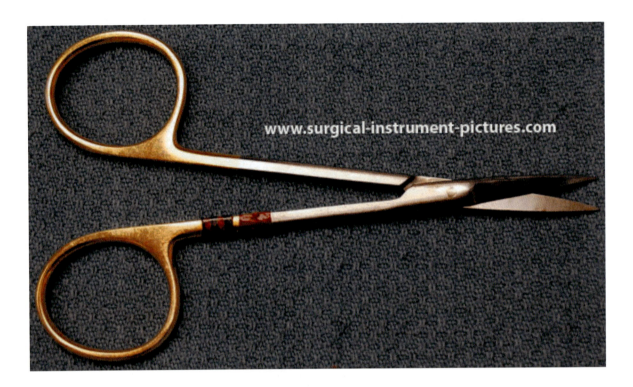

Surgical Instrument: Iris Scissors
Alias: None
Use: Cutting
Additional Info: Small scissors for sharp dissection of tissue

Nasal Rasp

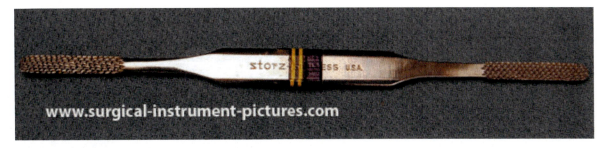

Surgical Instrument: Nasal Rasp
Alias: None
Use: Rasp
Additional Info: Rasp for Rhinoplasty Procedures

Strabismus Scissors

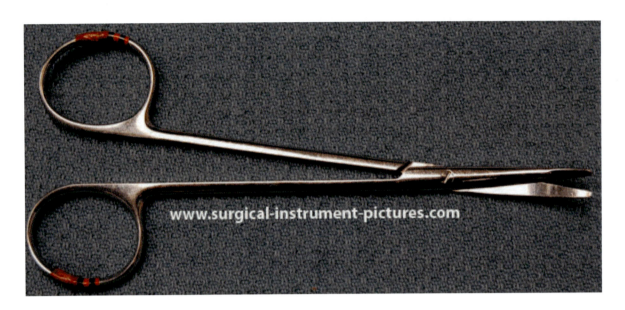

Surgical Instrument: Strabismus Scissors
Alias: Small Metz
Use: Cutting
Additional Info: Similar to but smaller than Metz Scissors

Stevens Tenotomy Scissors

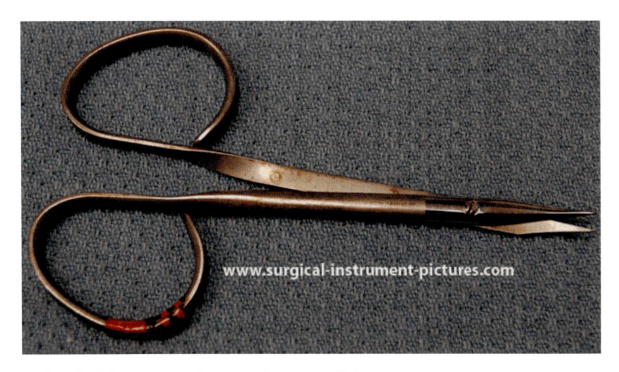

Surgical Instrument: Stevens Tenotomy Scissors
Alias: None
Use: Cutting
Additional Info: Very small fine sharp dissection scissors

Tenotomy Scissors

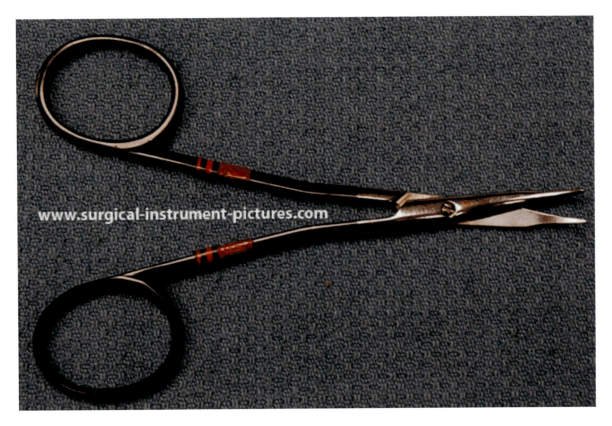

Surgical Instrument: Tenotomy Scissors
Alias: None
Use: Cutting
Additional Info: Fine razor-edged dissection scissors

Webster Needle Holder

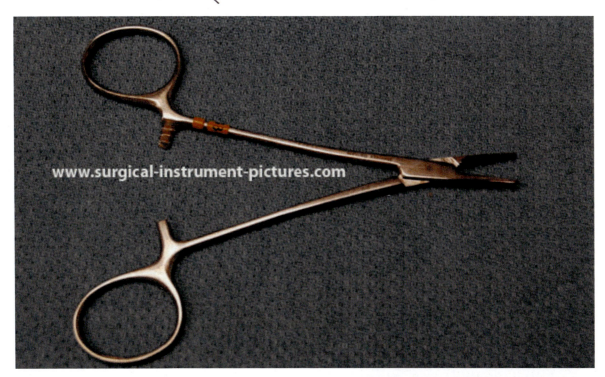

Surgical Instrument: Webster Needle Holder
Alias: None
Use: Suturing
Additional Info: Has a smooth jaw so as to not damage delicate suturing material

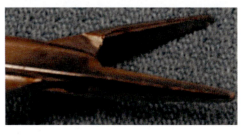

ENT Surgery

Adenoid Curette

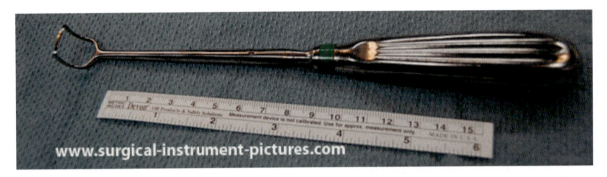

Surgical Instrument: Adenoid Curette
Alias: None
Use: Curetting
Additional Info: Used for ENT andenoid-ectomies

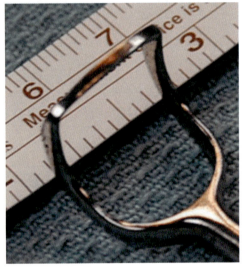

Angled Debakey

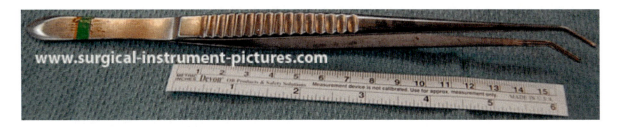

Surgical Instrument: Angled Debakey
Alias: None
Use: Grasping
Additional Info: Used for a tonsillectomy

Back Biting Through Cutting Forceps

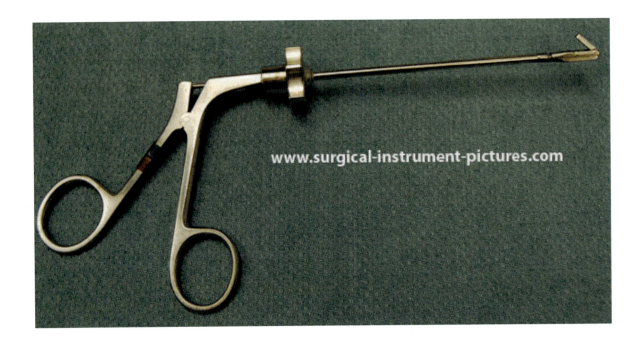

Surgical Instrument: Back Biting Forceps
Alias: Back Biter
Use: Cutting
Additional Info: Rotating head allows cutting tissue, bone and cartiage during sinus surgery

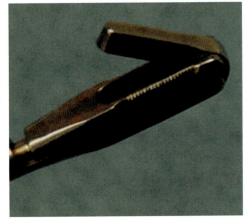

Cartilage Crusher

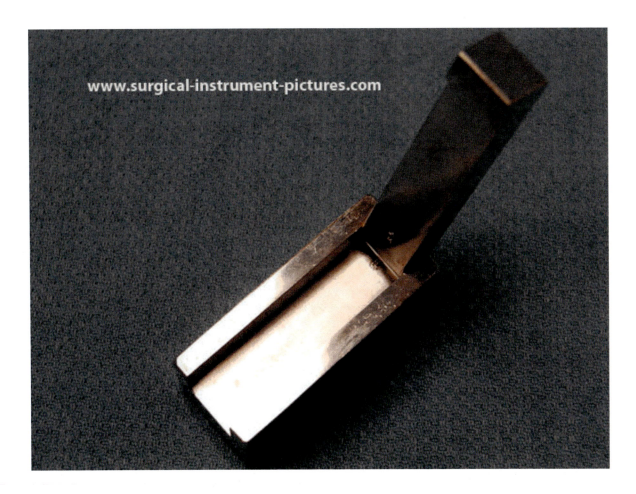

Surgical Instrument: Cartilage Crusher
Alias: None
Use: Crushing
Additional Info: Used for crushing cartilage for re-implantation during nose surgeries

Cartilage Block

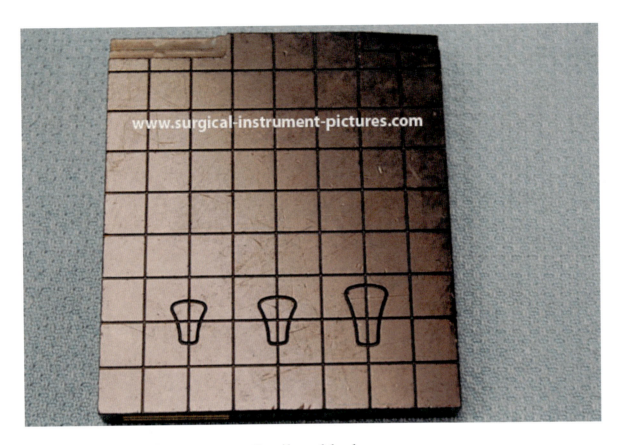

Surgical Instrument: Cartilage block
Alias: None
Use: Cutting surface
Additional Info: For preparation of grafts to be placed during rhinoplasty surgery

Cottle Elevator

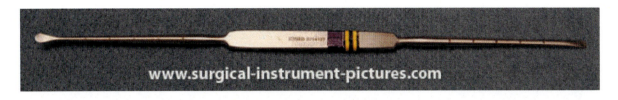

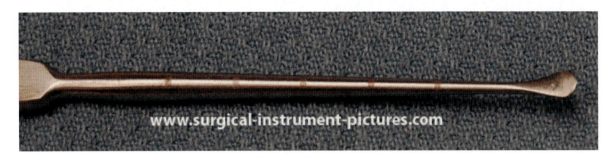

Surgical Instrument: Cottle Elevator
Alias: None
Use: Dissection
Additional Info: Common to ENT nasal sets

Curved Allis*

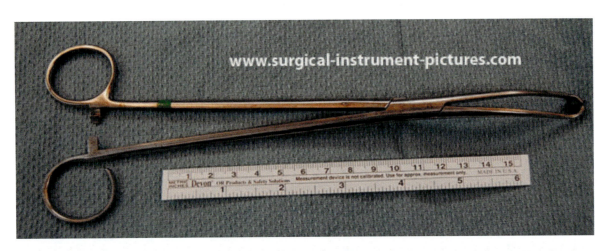

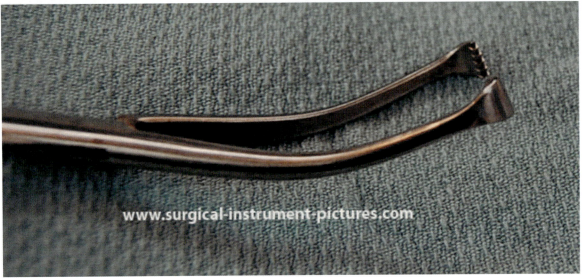

Surgical Instrument: Curved Allis
Alias: None
Use: Grasping
Additional Info: For grasping the tonsils during tonsillectomy

Up Biting Forceps

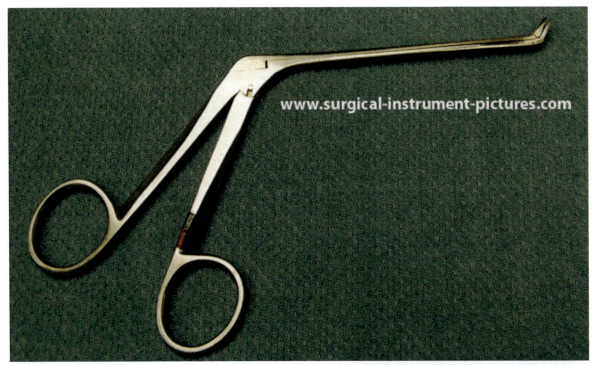

Surgical Instrument: Up biting forceps
Alias: None
Use: Grasping
Additional Info: Used for grasping and tearing during sinus and nasal surgery

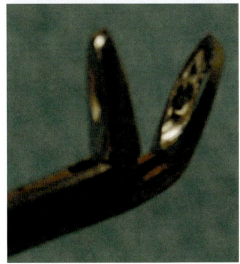

Davis Mouth Gag

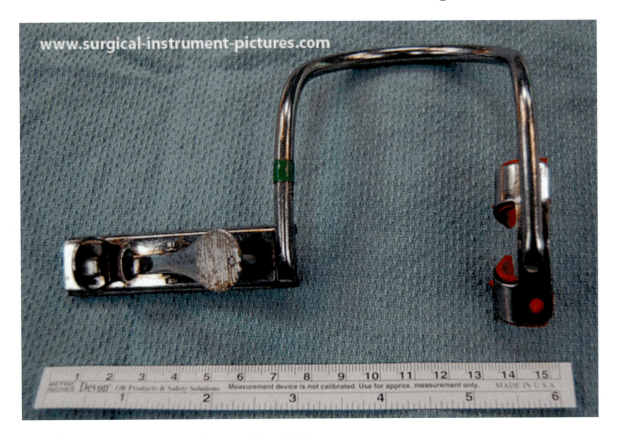

Surgical Instrument: Davis Mouth Gag
Alias: None
Use: Retraction
Additional Info: Attached to the mayo stand to hold the mouth open during a tonsillectomy

Tongue Blade for Mouth Gag

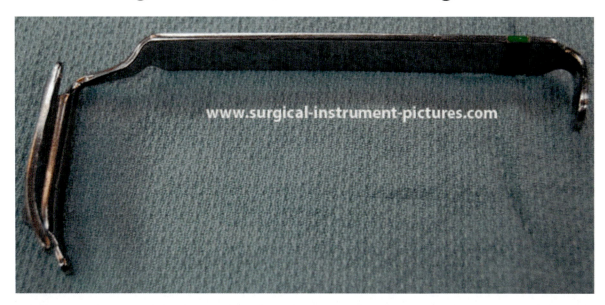

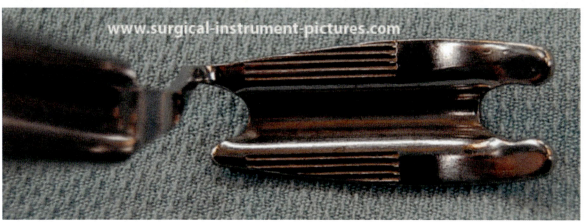

Surgical Instrument: Tongue Blade for Mouth Gag
Alias: None
Use: Retraction
Additional Info: Attaches to the Davis mouth gag to provide exposure for tonsil surgery

Mouth Gag Extension

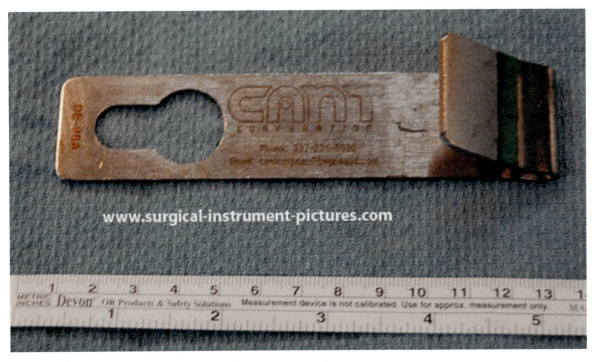

Surgical Instrument: Mouth gag extension
Alias: None
Use: Fixation
Additional Info: Attaches to the Mayo stand to extend the reach of the mouth gag in patients with a larger chest diameter

Sayer Elevator

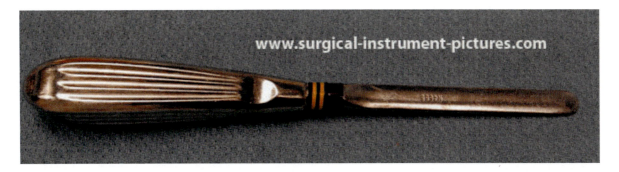

Surgical Instrument: Sayer Elevator
Alias: Butter Knife
Use: Breaking septal or nasal bone
Additional Info: None

Sinus Forceps

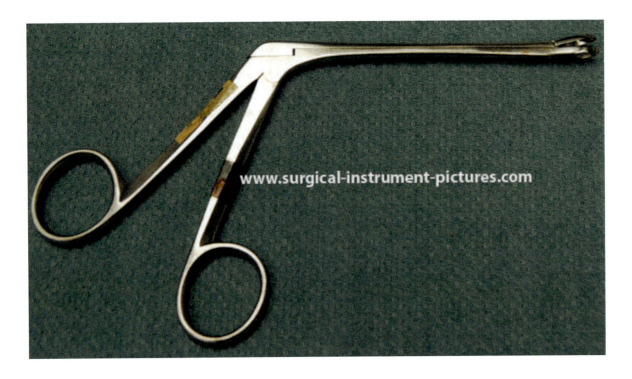

Surgical Instrument: Sinus Forceps
Alias: Straight Biter
Use: Grasping, cutting
Additional Info: Primary grasper for sinus surgery

Hurd Dissector

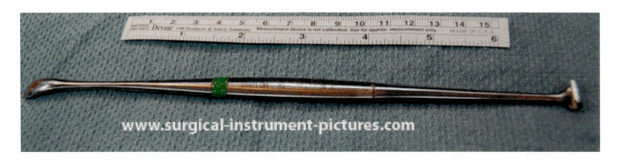

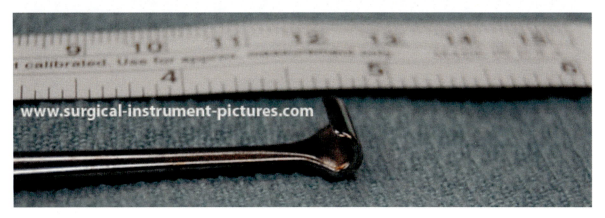

Surgical Instrument: Hurd Dissector
Alias: None
Use: Dissection
Additional Info: Blunt dissector/retractor for tonsil surgery

Sinus Scissors

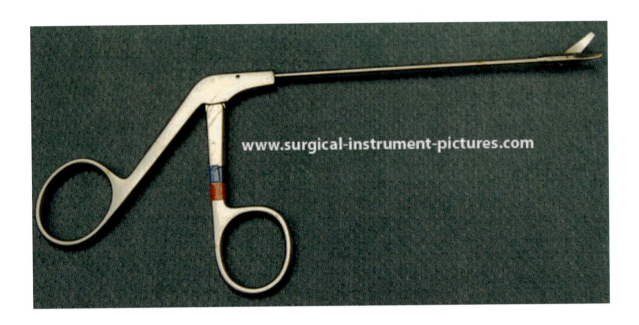

Surgical Instrument: Sinus Scissors
Alias: None
Use: Cutting
Additional Info: For cutting tissue within the sinus cavities

Frazier Suction Tip

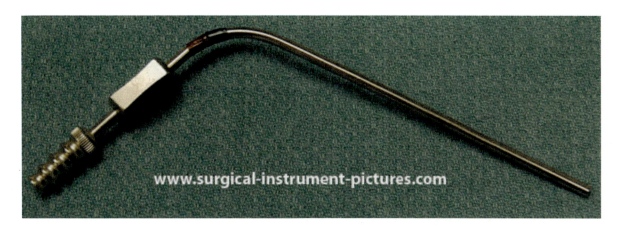

Surgical Instrument: Frazier Suction Tip
Alias: None
Use: Suction
Additional Info: Common to ENT and orthopedic surgery

Knight Scissors

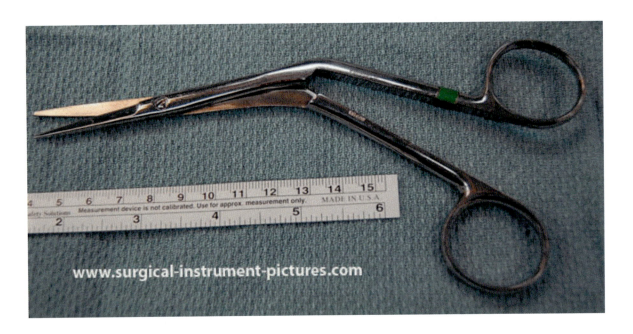

Surgical Instrument: Knight Scissors
Alias: None
Use: Cutting
Additional Info: Used for cutting tissue and suture within the nasal cavity.

~~Olive~~ Curved Tip Suction

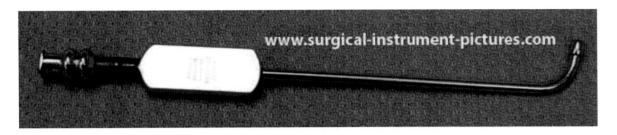

Surgical Instrument: Olive tip suction
Alias: None
Use: Suction
Additional Info: For suction within the sinus cavity

Sinus Probe

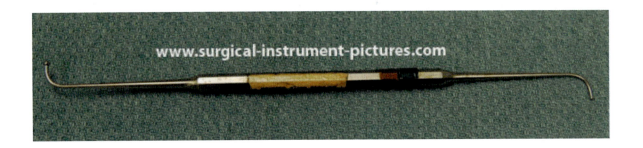

Surgical Instrument: Sinus Probe
Alias: Seeker
Use: Probing
Additional Info: For probing within the sinus cavity

Sickle Knife

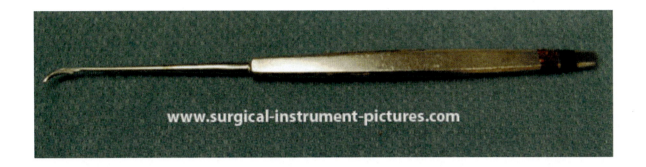

Surgical Instrument: Sickle knife
Alias: None
Use: Cutting
Additional Info: Non-disposable cutting blade for use in the sinus cavity

Sinus Currette

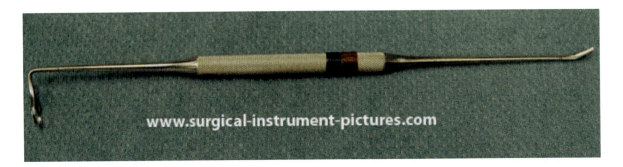

Surgical Instrument: Sinus Currette
Alias: None
Use: Curretting, scraping tissue
Additional Info: For curretting in the sinus cavity

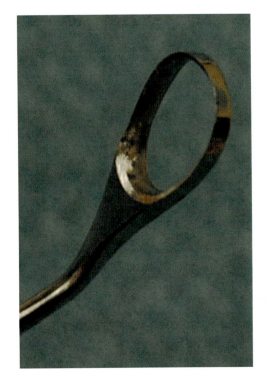

Giraffe Sphenoid Punch

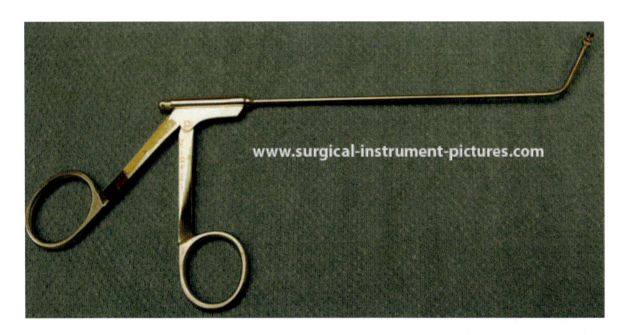

Surgical Instrument: Sphenoid Punch
Alias: None
Use: Cutting
Additional Info: Used to make a hole for access into the sphenoid sinus cavity

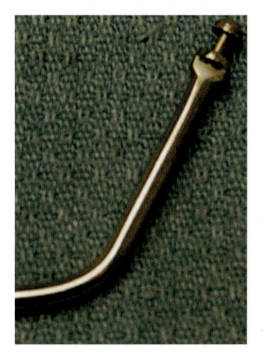

Sinus Biting Forcep

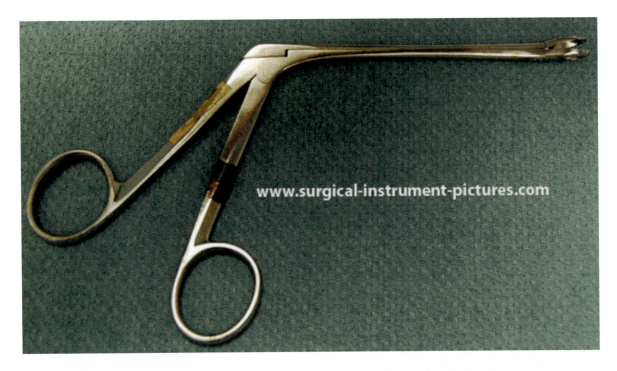

Surgical Instrument: Sinus Biting Forcep
Alias: None
Use: Grasping/Cutting
Additional Info: For cutting and grasping within the sinus cavities

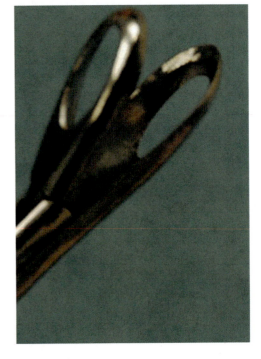

Takahashi Forceps

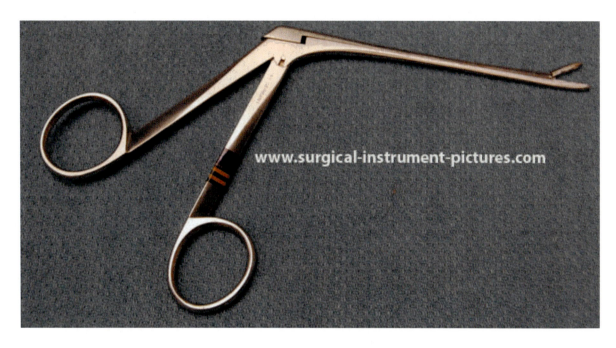

Surgical Instrument: Takahashi forceps
Alias: None
Use: Grasping
Additional Info: Common multipurpose ENT nasal/sinus grasper

Tonsil Snare

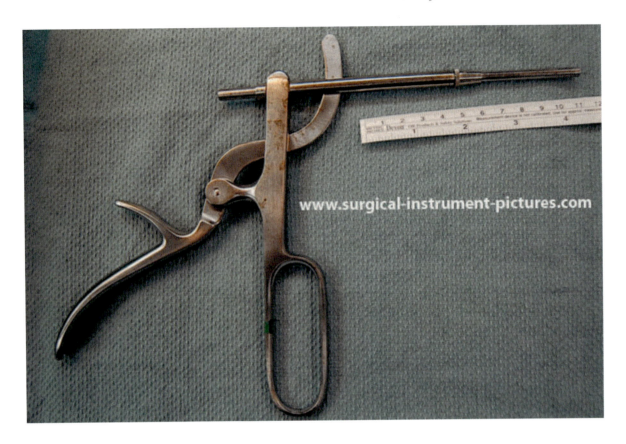

Surgical Instrument: Tonsil Snare
Alias: None
Use: Cutting
Additional Info: A wire snare extends from the barrel to encircle the tonsil and then retracts to cut the tonsil at the base. Not commonly used anymore because of other methods to cut and coagulate the bleeding at the same time

Nasal Speculum

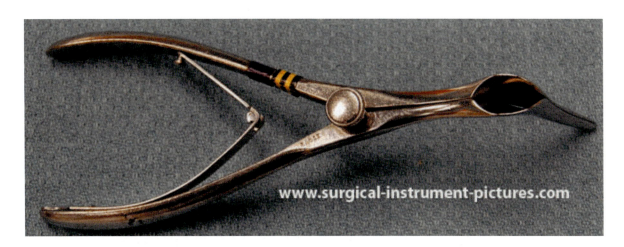

Surgical Instrument: Nasal Speculum
Alias: None
Use: retraction
Additional Info: Used to look up the nose

Weeder Tongue Blade

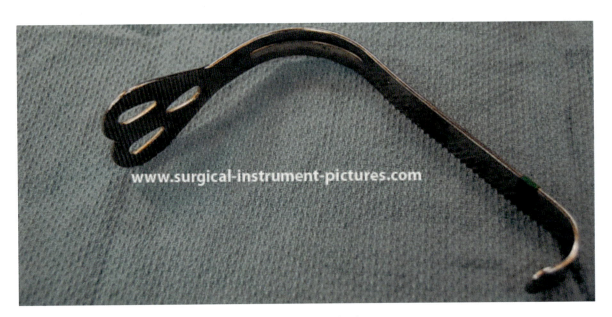

Surgical Instrument: Weeder Tongue Blade
Alias: None
Use: Retraction
Additional Info: For retraction of the tongue

Cottle Angular Scissors

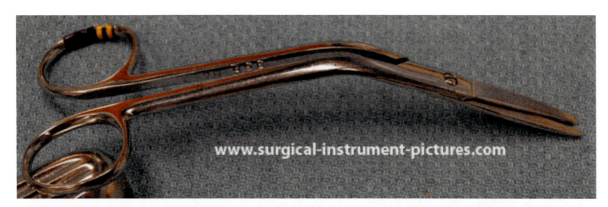

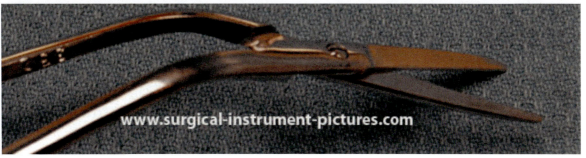

Surgical Instrument: Cottle Angular Scissors
Alias: None
Use: Cutting
Additional Info: For cutting inside the nasal cavity

INDEX

- #3 Knife Handle — 5
- #7 Knife Handle — 6
- 10 Blade — 2
- 11 Blade — 4
- 15 Blade — 3
- 90 Degree Dural Elevator — 97
- Adenoid Currette — 154
- Adson Bipolar Forceps — 44
- Adson Brown Forceps — 8
- Adson Forceps — 7
- Alexander Periosteotome — 65
- Allis Clamp — 13
- Alm Retractor — 130
- Angled Debakey — 155
- Aortic Clamp — 66
- AP Suction Tip — 64
- Army Navy Retractor — 23
- Babcock — 14
- Baby Bennett Retractor — 42
- Back Biting Forceps — 156
- Balfour Retractor — 128
- Bayonette Bipolar Forceps — 98
- Bayonette Forceps — 99
- Beaver Blade Handle — 43
- Bethune Rib Shears — 91
- Bishop Harmon Forceps — 131
- BoneTamp — 45
- Bonney Forceps — 9
- Bovie — 35
- Breast Template — 133
- Brun Currette — 46
- Burford Finochietto — 68
- Butter Knife — 165

- Caliper — 134
- Carmault — 15
- Cartilage Block — 158
- Cartilage Crusher — 157
- Castro Viejo Needle Holder — 71
- Cerebellar Retractor — 113
- Cherry Scissors — 100
- Cobb Elevator — 47
- Corneal Shield — 136
- Cottle Angular Scissors — 181
- Cottle Elevator — 159
- Curved Allis — 160
- Curved Dissector — 41
- Cushing Forceps — 101
- Davis Mouth Gag — 162
- Deaver Retractor — 24
- Debakey Clamp — 74-75
- Debakey Forceps — 10
- Demar Retractor — 137
- Detrich Forceps — 77
- Doyan Rib Rasp — 78
- Dural Retractor — 106
- Duval Lung Clamp — 82
- Electro Cautery Pencil — 35
- Facelift Scissors — 144
- Fiber Optic Breast Retractor — 141
- Fiber Optic Cord — 142
- Finochietto Blade — 68-69
- Fogarty Clamp — 83
- Four Pronged Skin Hooks — 145
- Frazier Suction Tip — 169
- Freeman Retractor — 143
- Freer Elevator — 49
- Gaurded Osteotome — 146
- Gelpi, Deep — 50

- Gelpi, Shallow — 103
- Gerald Forceps — 84
- Glover Clamp, Angled — 76
- Glover Clamp, Curved — 67
- Glover Clamp, Straight — 85
- Goelet Retractor — 26
- Hagar Scissors/Needle Holder — 132
- Heaney-Ballantine Clamp, Curved — 123
- Heaney-Ballantine Clamp, Straight — 122
- Heaney Needle Holder — 124
- Heaney-Simon Retractor — 119
- Hemo Clip Applier — 72
- Henley Retractor — 86
- Hoen Elevator — 52
- Hoke Osteotome — 53
- Hurd Dissector — 167
- Iris Scissors — 148
- Isreal Retractor — 27
- Jacob Tenaculm — 125
- Jake Clamp — 87
- Javid Carotid Clamp — 70
- Jorgenson Scissors — 120
- Karchner Internal Carotid Clamp — 80
- Kelly Clamp — 16
- Kerrison Rongeur — 104
- Key Elevator — 54
- Klein Needle — 140
- Knight Scissors — 170
- Kocher Clamp — 55
- K-Wire Cutter — 48
- Lahey Clamp — 126
- Lambotte Osteotome — 56
- Laparoscopic Grasper — 40
- Laparoscopic Port — 39
- Laparoscopic Trocar — 39

- Laparoscopic Trocar — 39
- Liposuction Cannula — 139
- Littler Scissors — 138
- Maryland Grasper — 41
- Mayo Bodywall Retractor — 28
- Mayo Scissors, Curved — 32
- Mayo Scissors, Straight — 31
- Mayo-Hegar Needle Holder — 38
- Metz — 34
- Metzenbaum Scissors — 34
- Mosquito Clamp — 17
- Mouth Gag Extension — 164
- Mouth Gag Tongue Blade — 163
- Nasal Rasp — 149
- Nasal Speculum — 179
- Nerve Hook — 105
- New York Speculum — 118
- Non-Perforating Towel Clamp — 22
- Olive Tip Suction — 171
- Penfield 1 — 107
- Penfield 2 — 108
- Penfield 3 — 109
- Penfield 4 — 110
- Perforating Towel Clamp — 21
- Pituitary Forceps — 112
- Poole Suction — 36
- Potts Scissors — 89
- Putti Rasp — 57
- Ragnell Retractor — 51
- Rainey Forceps — 58
- Rat Tooth Forceps — 11
- Rib Approximator — 90
- Richardson Retractor — 29
- Right Angle Clamp — 18
- Rongeur, Single Action — 59

- Rongeur, Double Action — 60
- Rummel Stylet — 92
- Russian Forceps — 12
- Sauerburch Retractor — 61
- Sauerbruch Rongeur — 94
- Scapula Retractor — 79
- Senn Retractor — 25
- Sickle Knife — 173
- Sims Retractor — 117
- Sinus Biting Forceps — 176
- Sinus Currette — 174
- Sinus Forceps — 166
- Sinus Probe — 172
- Sinus Scissors — 168
- Sphenoid Punch — 175
- Sponge Forceps — 19
- Spring Retractor — 62
- Statinsky Clamp — 88
- Statinsky Scissors — 93
- Stevens Tenotomy Scissors — 151
- Strabismus Scissors — 150
- T Clamp — 127
- Takahashi Forceps — 177
- Tenaculum, Double Tooth — 115
- Tendon Passer — 63
- Tenotomy Scissors — 152
- Tonsil Clamp — 20
- Tonsil Snare — 178
- Two Pronge Skin Hooks — 147
- Up Biting Forceps — 161
- Uterine Sound — 129
- Vein Retractor — 73
- Vessel Irrigator — 95
- Vessel Probe — 96
- Webster Needle Holder — 153

- Weeder Tongue Blade   180
- Weighted Vaginal Speculum   116
- Weitlaner Retractor, Dull   30
- Weitlaner Retractor, Sharp   31
- Westcott Scissors   135
- Woodson Elevator   114
- Wylie External Carotid Clamp   81
- Yankauer Suction   37

Made in the USA
Las Vegas, NV
16 December 2021

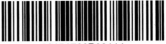